Heart Healthy Cookbook After 50

2 Books in 1: 100+ Fuss-Free, Delicious Recipes that are Low Sodium and Easy to Prepare

Julieth Kern

indirect, which are incurred as a result of the use of information contained within this document, including, but not limited to, errors, omissions, or inaccuracies.

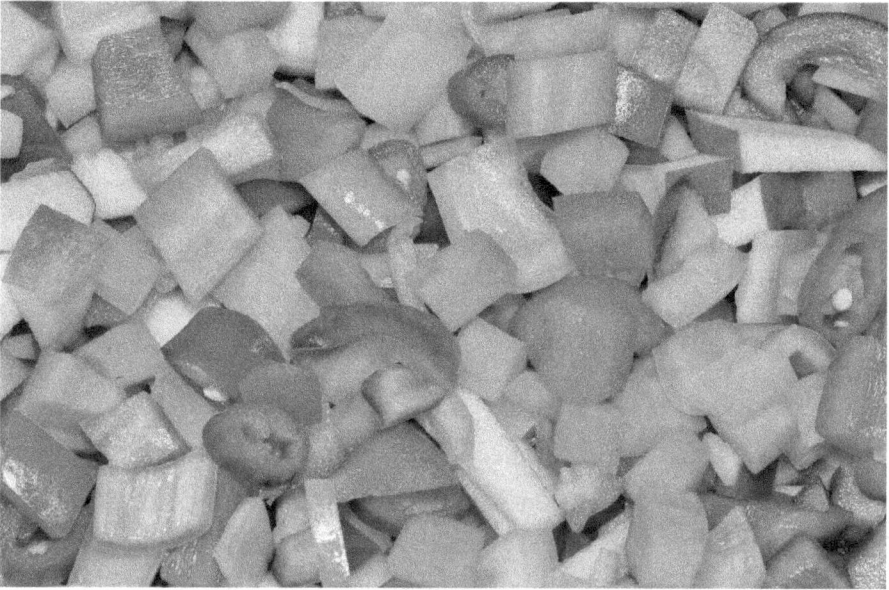

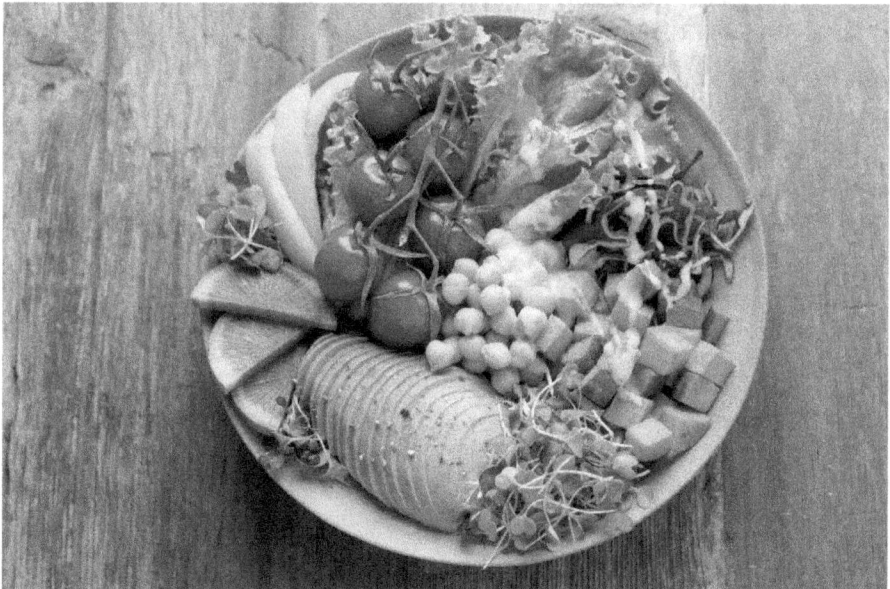

Table of Contents

APPETIZERS, SNACKS, AND PARTY FOODS..........10

1 HOT PECAN DIP 11
2 PECAN CHEESE WAFERS..........13
3 MACADAMIA CHEESE CRISPS 14
4 BARBECUED NUTS 15
5 SPICY PECANS 16
6 SPICY NUT MIX 17
7 PARTY NUT MIX..........18
8 SUGARED PECANS 19

BREAKFAST 21

9 CALIFORNIA BREAKFAST SANDWICH 21
10 EASY BREAKFAST STRATA 23
11 APPLE PANCAKES 24
12 HIGH-PROTEIN BLUEBERRY PANCAKES 25
13 PRALINE FRENCH TOAST 26
14 BANANA PUMPKIN MUFFINS 28
15 BLUEBERRY OATMEAL MUFFINS 30

MAIN DISHES..........32

16 OLD-FASHIONED VEGETABLE SOUP..........32
17 PUMPKIN SOUP..........34
18 PUMPKIN VEGETABLE SOUP 35
19 TOMATO VEGETABLE SOUP 36
20 VEGETABLE PASTA SAUCE 38
21 BEEF, BEAN, AND CABBAGE STEW 39
22 MEXICAN BEEF SALAD..........40
23 MEXICAN SPAGHETTI PIE 41
24 SOUTHWESTERN VEGETABLE STEW..........43
25 ITALIAN OVEN CHOWDER 45
26 TACO SALAD 46
27 TEXAS CORNBREAD SKILLET MEAL 47
28 CHICKEN AND BLACK BEANS 49

SIDE DISHES AND SALADS..........51

29 POTATO DUMPLINGS..........51
30 POTATO AND VEGETABLE HASH 53
31 AVOCADO AND CRABMEAT SALAD 54
32 BROCCOLI AND TOMATO SALAD 55
33 BROCCOLI CAULIFLOWER SALAD 57

34 CABBAGE FRUIT SALAD 58
35 CORN SALAD 59
36 DATE APPLE WALDORF SALAD 60
37 FIESTA SALAD 61
38 GRAPEFRUIT, AVOCADO, AND SPINACH SALAD 63
39 ORANGE AVOCADO SALAD 65
40 SPNACH AND ORANGE SECTION SALAD 66

BREADS **67**

41 MULTIGRAIN ROLLS 67
42 RYE ROLLS 69
43 FOCACCIA ROLLS 70

DESSERTS AND OTHER SWEETS **72**

44 CRUNCHY ORANGE COOKIES 72
45 FRUIT COOKIES 74
46 GRAHAM CRACKER PRALINE COOKIES 75
47 GRANOLA COOKIES 76
48 RAISIN-GRANOLA COOKIES 77
49 PECAN COOKIES 79
50 PEANUT-GRANOLA COOKIES 81

APPETIZERS, SNACKS, AND PARTY FOODS **85**

1 PARMESAN-GARLIC PITA TOASTS 85
2 SPICY PITA DIPPERS 87
3 WHOLE WHEAT HONEY MUSTARD PRETZELS 88
4 RANCH-STYLE PRETZELS 89
5 CAJUN PARTY MIX 90
6 CURRIED SNACK MIX 91
7 S'MORE SNACK MIX 92
8 CARAMEL CORN 93

BREAKFAST **95**

9   CINNAMON HONEY SCONES 95
10 OATMEAL RAISIN SCONES 97
11 WHOLE GRAIN SCONES 98
12 GRANOLA 100
13 TOASTY NUT GRANOLA 101
14 BREAKFAST BARS 102
15 WHOLE WHEAT COFFEE CAKE 104

MAIN DISHES **107**

16 CHICKEN CHILI VERDE 107

17   PORK CHOP AND BEAN SKILLET 109
18   BEAN BALLS.. 110
19   CHICKPEA SANDWICH SPREAD 111
20   ITALIAN BAKED BEANS 112
21   WHITE BEAN AND TUNA SALAD 114
22   BEEF AND BARLEY STEW 115
23   BEEF BARLEY SKILLET 117
24   STROGANOFF 118
25   WESTERN CASSEROLE 119
26   CHICKEN BARLEY CHOWDER 120
27   CHICKEN BARLEY SOUP.. 121
28   CHICKEN CHILI WITH BARLEY 122

SIDE DISHES AND SALADS... 124
29   MEXICAN RICE 124
30   TOMATO PILAF 125
31   RICE AND CHEESE CASSEROLE 126
32   SOUTHERN RICE PILAF 127
33   BARLEY AND PINE NUT CASSEROLE... 129
34   BARLEY CASSEROLE 130
35   BARLEY MUSHROOM PILAF 131
36   BARLEY RISOTTO... 132
37   BULGUR PILAF 133
38   BULGUR WHEAT WITH SQUASH 134
39   STUFFED TOMATOES... 135
40   RIGATONI WITH ARTICHOKE SAUCE... 137

BREADS... 138
41   MAPLE OATMEAL BREAD 138
42   GERMAN DARK BREAD 140
43   ONION AND GARLIC WHEAT BREAD 141

DESSERTS AND OTHER SWEETS 143
44   GRANOLA BARS 143
45   HONEY OATMEAL CAKE 145
46   RED VELVET CAKE 147
47   BROWN RICE PUDDING 149
48   COOL RICE 150
49   WHOLE WHEAT PIECRUST... 151
50   HIGH-FIBER PIECRUST 152

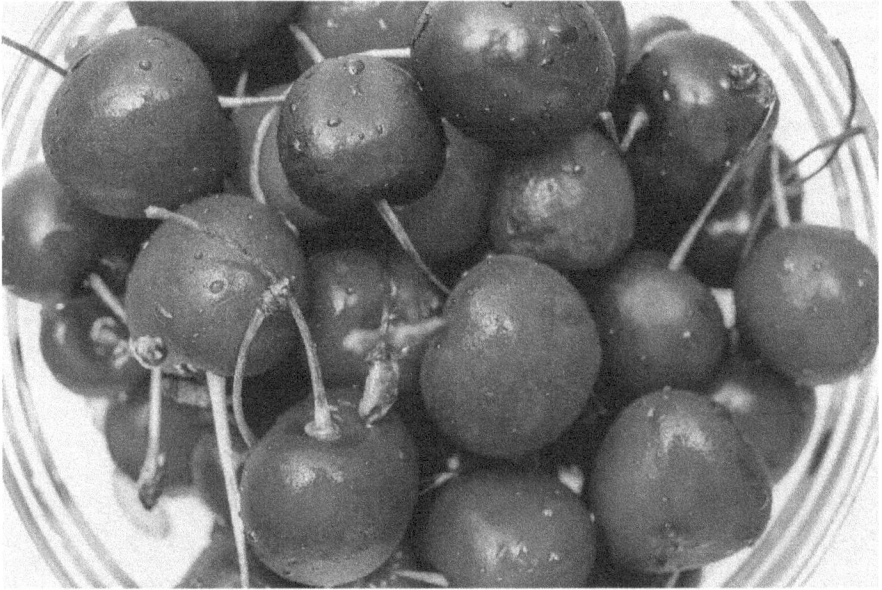

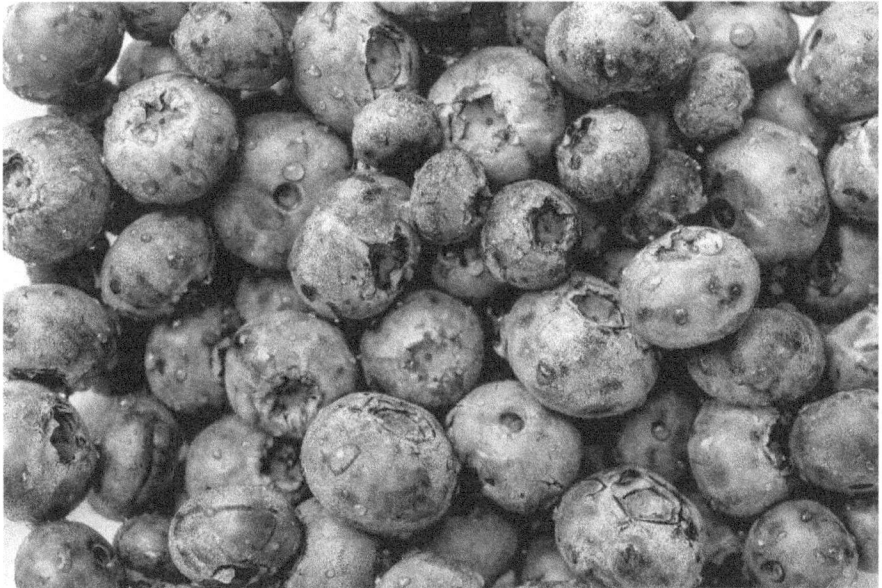

Heart Healthy Cookbook for Beginners 2021

50+ Fuss-Free, Delicious Recipes that are Low Sodium and Easy to Prepare

Julieth Kern

Appetizers, Snacks, and Party Foods

We'll start our trip with appetizers and snack foods and begin that journey with legumes. The first thing that probably comes to mind is bean dip. We have five different bean dips, and you'll also find dips and spreads using less common legumes such as black-eyed peas and chick peas. There are also a number of other items like salsa, nachos, stuffed eggs and one of my new personal favorites, roasted chickpeas.

1 Hot Pecan Dip

Dried beef and toasted pecans provide the flavor here.

cu^2/₃ (74 g) pecans, toasted

1 tablespoons (28 g) unsalted butter

8 ounces (225 g) cream cheese

½ cup (115 g) sour cream

¼ teaspoon garlic powder

¼ teaspoon black pepper

½ cup (8O g) grated onion

¼ cup (C8 g) chopped green bell pepper C ounces (85 g) chopped dried beef

Toast pecans in butter. Cream together remaining ingredients. Spread creamed mixture in buttered 9-inch (23 cm) pie plate. Top with toasted pecans and bake 20 minutes in 350°F (180°C, gas mark 4) oven.

Yield: 12 servings

Each with: 32 g water; 153 calories (81% from fat, 12% from protein, 7% from carb); 5 g protein;
14 g total fat; 7 g saturated fat; 5 g monounsaturated fat; 2 g polyunsaturated fat; 3 g carb; 1 g fiber; 1
g sugar; 63 mg phosphorus; 33 mg calcium; 1 mg iron; 258 mg

sodium; 98 mg potassium; 366 IU vitamin A; 94 mg vitamin E; 3 mg vitamin C; 35 mg cholesterol

2 Pecan Cheese Wafers

These savory little pecan and cheese crackers are great to snack on or asdippers.

½ cup (112 g) unsalted butter, softened 2 cups (225 g) shredded Cheddar cheese 1 cup (11O g) finely chopped pecans

1 cup (12O g) whole wheat pastry flour

¼ teaspoon cayenne pepper

Cream butter and cheese. Add pecans, flour, and cayenne. Mix well. Form into 2 rolls, 1-inch (2.5 cm) diameter. Wrap in plastic and refrigerate severalhours or overnight. (This can also be frozen.) Slice rolls into thin rounds and place on baking sheet coated with nonstick vegetable oil spray. Bake at 350°F (180°C, gas mark 4) for 15 minutes or until edges brown lightly. Remove to a rack to cool.

Yield: 40 servings

Each with: 3 g water; 76 calories (75% from fat, 12% from protein, 13% from carb); 2 g protein; 7 g total fat; 3 g saturated fat; 2 g monounsaturated fat; 1 g polyunsaturated fat; 3 g carb; 1 g fiber; 0 g sugar; 52 mg phosphorus; 51 mg calcium; 0 mg iron; 41 mg sodium; 31 mg potassium; 143 IUvitamin A; 36 mg vitamin E; 0 mg vitamin C; 13 mg cholesterol

3 Macadamia Cheese Crisps

These savory little crackers have the added bonus of macadamia nuts. You'll find it hard to limit yourself to the recommended serving size.

½ cup (112 g) unsalted butter

¼ pound (115 g) grated Swiss cheese1 egg
1½ cups (18O g) whole wheat pastry flourcup (45 g) chopped macadamia nuts

Preheat oven to 400°F (200°C, gas mark 6). Blend butter, cheese, and egg. Gradually work in flour and nuts. Mold into a roll 1½ inches (4 cm) in diameter. Wrap in waxed paper and chill until firm. Slice dough into ¼-inch (0.5 cm) slices. Place on lightly buttered baking sheet and bake for 10 to 15 minutes or until lightly browned.

Yield: 18 servings

Each with: 6 g water; 126 calories (64% from fat, 12% from protein, 24% from carb); 4 g protein; 9 g total fat; 5 g saturated fat; 3 g monounsaturated fat; 0 g polyunsaturated fat; 8 g carb; 1 g fiber; 0 g sugar; 84 mg phosphorus; 69 mg calcium; 1 mg iron; 7 mg sodium; 62 mg potassium; 229 IUvitamin A; 61 mg vitamin E; 0 mg vitamin C; 31 mg cholesterol

4 Barbecued Nuts

These are not your usual nuts. The flavor and spiciness can be varied depending on what kind of barbecue sauce you use.

4 cups (58O g) mixed nuts

1 cup (25O g) barbecue sauce

2 tablespoons grated Parmesan cheese

Heat oven to 300°F (150°C, gas mark 2). In medium bowl, combine mixed nuts and barbecue sauce; stir until evenly coated. Spread on ungreased baking sheet; sprinkle with Parmesan cheese. Bake at 350°F (180°C, gas mark 4) for 20 to 25 minutes or until nuts are dry. Transfer to waxed paper. Cool completely. Store in tightly covered container.

Yield: 16 servings

Each with: 10 g water; 254 calories (68% from fat, 10% from protein, 23% from carb); 6 g protein; 20 g total fat; 3 g saturated fat; 11 g monounsaturated fat; 5 g polyunsaturated fat; 15 g carb; 3 gfiber; 7 g sugar; 170 mg phosphorus; 47 mg calcium; 1 mg iron; 312 mg sodium; 207 mg potassium; 6 IU vitamin A; 1 mg vitamin E; 0 mg vitamin C; 1 mg cholesterol

5 Spicy Pecans

Tabasco adds a little heat to these pecans.

2 tablespoons (28 g) unsalted butter

½ teaspoon salt-free seasoning blend (such as Mrs. Dash)teaspoon Tabasco sauce

1 pound (455 g) pecan halves

C tablespoons (45 ml) Worcestershire sauce

Put butter, seasoning, and Tabasco sauce in 12 × 8 × 2-inch (30 × 20 × 5- cm) baking dish. Place in 300°F (150°C, gas mark 2) oven until buttermelts. Add pecans, stirring until all are coated with butter. Bake for about 15 minutes, stirring occasionally. Sprinkle with Worcestershire sauce and stir again. Continue baking another 10 minutes until crisp.

Yield: 12 servings

Each with: 3 g water; 281 calories (87% from fat, 5% from protein, 8% from carb); 4 g protein; 29 g total fat; 4 g saturated fat; 16 g monounsaturated fat; 8 g polyunsaturated fat; 6 g carb; 4 g fiber; 2 g sugar; 109 mg phosphorus; 27 mg calcium; 1 mg iron; 37 mg sodium; 186 mg potassium; 85 IUvitamin A; 16 mg vitamin E; 7 mg vitamin C; 5 mg cholesterol

6 Spicy Nut Mix

Unlike the cinnamon-sugar nuts in this chapter, these are chili spiced,providing a savory snack.

1¼ cups (175 g) cashews

¾ cup (1O9 g) soy nuts

1 cup (145 g) sunflower seeds

2 tablespoons (28 ml) canola oil1½ teaspoons chili powder

   te⅛poon garlic powder

1 teaspoon Worcestershire sauce

Combine nuts and seeds in large bowl. Place oil, spices, and Worcestershiresauce in covered container. Cover and shake. Sprinkle over nuts and seeds. Toss to coat. Spread in baking pan. Bake 20 minutes at 300°F (150°C, gas mark 2). Cool and store in covered containers in refrigerator.

Yield: 16 servings

Each with: 0 g water; 161 calories (66% from fat, 15% from protein, 19% from carb); 6 g protein;
12 g total fat; 2 g saturated fat; 5 g monounsaturated fat; 5 g polyunsaturated fat; 8 g carb; 2 g fiber; 1
g sugar; 198 mg phosphorus; 22 mg calcium; 1 mg iron; 8 mg sodium; 246 mg potassium; 71 IU vitamin A; 0 mg vitamin E; 1 mg vitamin C; 0 mg cholesterol

7 Party Nut Mix

Basically a sweet and spicy variation on the traditional cereal mix, this oneis mostly nuts.

8 ounces (225 g) dry-roasted peanuts

8 ounces (225 g) dry-roasted cashews 6 ounces (17O g) almonds

2 cups (6O g) square wheat cereal, such as Wheat Chex ¼ cup (55 g) unsalted butter, melted 1½ tablespoons (22 ml) soy sauce

1½ tablespoons (22 ml) Worcestershire sauce

¼ teaspoon Tabasco sauce1 cup (145 g) raisins
Combine first 4 ingredients in a large bowl; stir well. Combine butter, soy sauce, Worcestershire sauce, and Tabasco; mix well and pour over nutmixture, tossing to coat. Spread half of mixture in a 15 × 10 × 1-inch (37 × 25 × 2.5 cm) jelly-roll pan. Bake at 325°F (170°C, gas mark 3) for 15 minutes; cool and place in a large bowl. Repeat with remaining mixture. Add raisins and stir well. Store in an airtight container. **Yield:** 28 servings

Each with: 3 g water; 174 calories (61% from fat, 11% from protein, 28% from carb); 5 g protein; 13 g total fat; 3 g saturated fat; 7 g monounsaturated fat; 3 g polyunsaturated fat; 13 g carb; 2 g fiber; 5 g sugar; 118 mg phosphorus; 27 mg calcium; 2 mg iron; 66 mg sodium; 209 mg potassium; 60 IUvitamin A; 14 mg vitamin E; 3 mg vitamin C; 4 mg cholesterol

8 Sugared Pecans

These are sweet and just slightly spicy nuts. I came up with the recipe while on a search to duplicate the spiced nuts sold at places like the Maryland Renaissance Festival. They aren't quite the same, but they're closer than the baked ones.

¾ cup (15O g) sugar

2 teaspoons cinnamon

¼ cup (6O ml) water2 cups (22O g) pecans

Mix sugar and cinnamon in pan. Pour in water. Put in nuts. Bring to boil over medium heat; turn heat down and simmer, barely bubbling, 20 minutes or until syrup dries. Place nuts on waxed paper. Cool.

Yield: 12 servings

Each with: 6 g water; 176 calories (63% from fat, 4% from protein, 33% from carb); 2 g protein; 13 g total fat; 1 g saturated fat; 7 g monounsaturated fat; 4 g polyunsaturated fat; 15 g carb; 2 g fiber; 13 g sugar; 51 mg phosphorus; 18 mg calcium; 1 mg iron; 0 mg sodium; 77 mg potassium; 11 IU vitamin A; 0 mg vitamin E; 0 mg vitamin C; 0 mg cholesterol

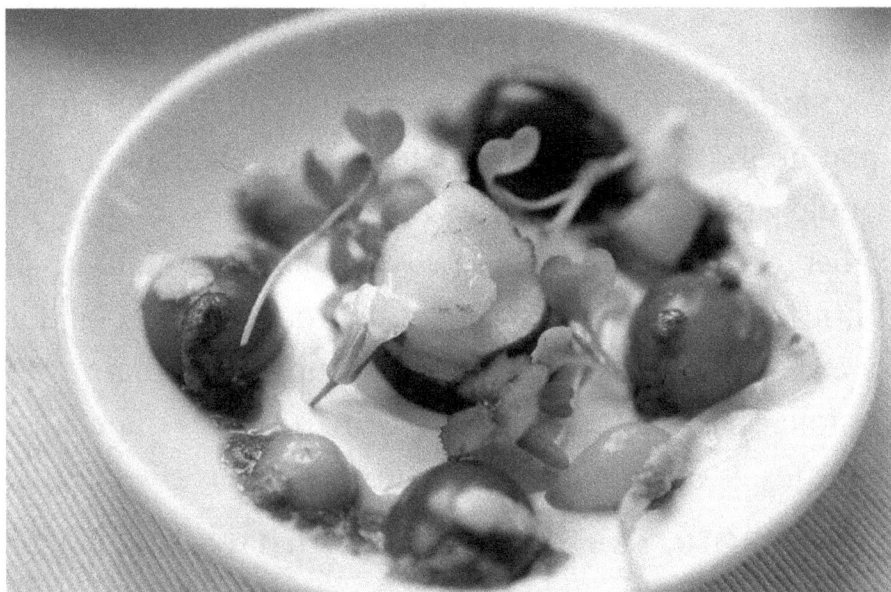

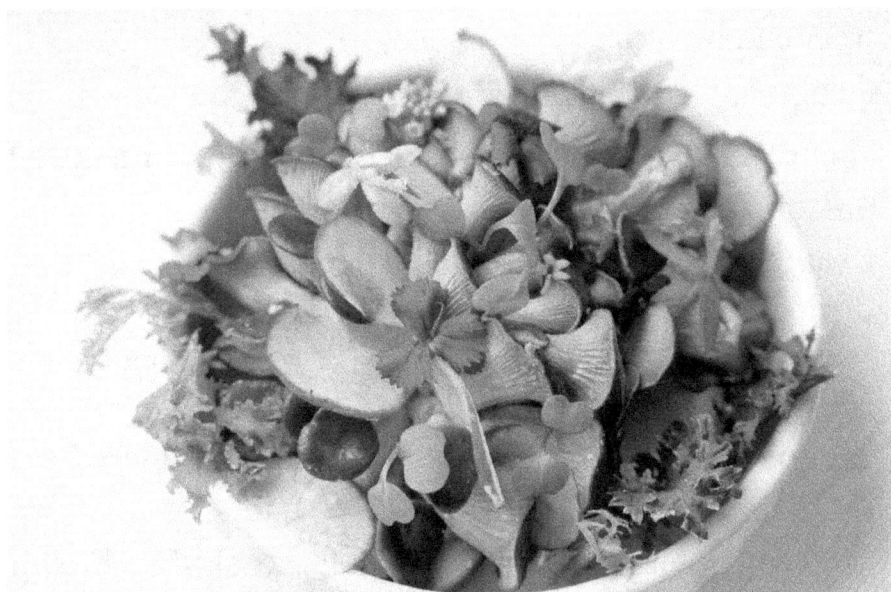

Breakfast

Breakfast is a key meal to get your day started right, and grains are a natural way to do that. Of course, you could choose the quick and easy solution of a high-fiber cereal. But sometimes you want something a little different. At least I know I do. In this chapter we have some ways to spice up your plain old oatmeal, as well as a variety of recipes for pancakes, waffles, scones, and homemade granola.

9 California Breakfast Sandwich

A Mexican version of eggs Benedict—this is a great weekend breakfast.

6 eggs

¾ cup (120 g) chopped onion1 tablespoon unsalted butter

2 ounces (55 g) mushrooms, sliced

1 avocado, sliced

½ cup (90 g) chopped tomato

½ cup (60 g) grated Cheddar cheese6 whole wheat English muffins

Mix eggs with wire whisk. In large skillet, brown onion with butter until clear and limp. Add mushrooms, avocado, and tomato. Stir. Add beaten eggs. Cook until almost set; add grated cheese. Spoon onto toasted English muffins.

Yield: 6 servings

Each with: 126 g water; 319 calories (43% from fat, 19% from protein, 37% from carb); 16 g protein; 16 g total fat; 6 g saturated fat; 6 g monounsaturated fat; 2 g polyunsaturated fat; 31 g carb; 5 g fiber; 3 g sugar; 254 mg phosphorus; 220 mg calcium; 3 mg iron; 368 mg sodium; 396 mg potassium; 581 IU vitamin A; 122 mg vitamin E; 5 mg vitamin C; 254 mg cholesterol

10 Easy Breakfast Strata

This is another great fix-ahead breakfast. We usually have some variation of this on special holidays when there is a lot to do in the morning, but we want a special family breakfast.

1 pound (455 g) sausage

8 eggs 1O slices whole wheat bread, cubed C cups (71O g) skim milk 2 cups (225 g) shredded Cheddar cheese 1O ounces (28O g) frozen chopped broccoli, thawed 2 tablespoons (28 g) unsalted butter, melted 2 tablespoons (16 g) flour1 tablespoon dry mustard2 teaspoons basil

In large skillet, brown sausage and drain. In large bowl, beat eggs. Add remaining ingredients and mix well. Spoon into 13 × 9-inch (33 × 23 cm) baking pan coated with nonstick vegetable oil spray. Cover and refrigerate 8 hours or overnight. Preheat oven to 350°F (180°C, gas mark 4). Bake 60 to 70 minutes or until knife inserted near center comes out clean.

Yield: 8 servings

Each with: 181 g water; 379 calories (49% from fat, 25% from protein, 26% from carb); 24 g protein; 21 g total fat; 11 g saturated fat; 6 g monounsaturated fat; 2 g polyunsaturated fat; 24 g carb; 2 g fiber; 3 g sugar; 449 mg phosphorus; 462 mg calcium; 3 mg iron; 593 mg sodium; 396 mg potassium; 1293 IU vitamin A; 243 mg vitamin E; 15 mg vitamin C; 281 mg cholesterol

11 Apple Pancakes

This makes a great breakfast for a weekend (or maybe when you aresnowed in). They're kind of like apple fritters, only the syrup flavor gets baked right into the pancakes.

4 cups (44O g) sliced apple ½ cup (12O ml) maple syrup 2 tablespoons (28 g) unsalted butter1½ cups (192 g) biscuit baking mix 1 cup (2C5 ml) skim milk 2 eggs ½ teaspoon cinnamon

¼ teaspoon nutmeg

Combine apples in skillet with syrup and butter. Cook until tender but firm, about 25 minutes. Meanwhile combine rest of ingredients and mix until smooth. Remove apples from skillet with slotted spoon and add to batter. Fold gently until apples are covered. Lift batter-covered apples onto hot griddle coated with nonstick vegetable oil spray. Grill until edges are cooked. Turn pancakes once. Serve with remaining syrup in which apples were cooked.

Yield: 6 servings

Each with: 126 g water; 306 calories (30% from fat, 8% from protein, 62% from carb); 7 g protein; 10 g total fat; 4 g saturated fat; 4 g monounsaturated fat; 1 g polyunsaturated fat; 48 g carb; 2 g fiber; 27 g sugar; 258 mg phosphorus; 145 mg calcium; 2 mg iron; 417 mg sodium; 269 mg potassium; 323 IU vitamin A; 83 mg vitamin E; 4 mg vitamin C; 91 mg cholesterol

12 High-Protein Blueberry Pancakes

When you are looking for a great-tasting breakfast but want something that also is good for you, you should give these pancakes a try.

4 eggs

1 cup (225 g) cottage cheese

¼ cup (28 g) wheat germ

¼ cup (20 g) quick-cooking oats 2 tablespoons (28 ml) canola oil

1 cup (145 g) blueberries

Place all the ingredients except blueberries in a blender and mix thoroughly. Stir in blueberries. Drop by tablespoons onto a hot frying pan or griddle coated with nonstick vegetable oil spray.

Yield: 4 servings

Each with: 103 g water; 240 calories (51% from fat, 27% from protein, 22% from carb); 16 g protein; 14 g total fat; 3 g saturated fat; 7 g monounsaturated fat; 3 g polyunsaturated fat; 13 g carb; 2 g fiber; 5 g sugar; 254 mg phosphorus; 49 mg calcium; 2 mg iron; 84 mg sodium; 200 mg potassium; 311 IU vitamin A; 81 mg vitamin E; 4 mg vitamin C; 239 mg cholesterol

13 Praline French Toast

This breakfast treat is like a taste of old New Orleans and will definitely beon your list to make again.

8 eggs

1½ cups (C55 ml) skim milk

½ cup (115 g) brown sugar, divided 2 teaspoons vanilla extract

8 slices whole wheat bread

¼ cup (55 g) unsalted butter

¼ cup (6O ml) maple syrup

½ cup (55 g) chopped pecans

Thoroughly blend eggs, milk, 1 tablespoon brown sugar, and vanilla. Pour half of egg mixture into 9 × 13-inch (23 × 33 cm) baking dish. Place bread slices in mixture. Pour remaining egg mixture over bread. Cover and refrigerate several hours or overnight. Preheat oven to 350°F (180°C, gas mark 4). Remove bread from baking dish and set aside. Place butter in 9 × 13-inch (23 × 33-cm) baking dish and put in oven until butter melts. Stir in remaining brown sugar and syrup. Sprinkle with pecans. Carefully place reserved bread slices on pecans. Pour any remaining egg mixture overbread. Bake uncovered until puffed and lightly brown, 30 to 35 minutes. Invert slices to serve.

Yield: 8 servings

Each with: 98 g water; 345 calories (45% from fat, 14% from protein, 41% from carb); 12 g protein; 17 g total fat; 6 g saturated fat; 7 g monounsaturated fat; 3 g polyunsaturated fat; 36 g carb; 2 g fiber; 22 g sugar; 221 mg phosphorus; 156 mg calcium; 2 mg iron; 243 mg sodium; 304 mg potassium; 547 IU vitamin A; 154 mg vitamin E; 1 mg vitamin C; 253 mg cholesterol

14 Banana Pumpkin Muffins

These moist pumpkin muffins have a spiced brown sugar topping.

½ cup (112 g) pureed banana

½ cup (12C g) canned pumpkin

½ cup (1OO g) sugar

¼ cup (6O ml) skim milk

¼ cup (6O ml) canola oil1 egg
1¾ cups (21O g) whole wheat pastry flour 2 teaspoons baking powder
1 teaspoon pumpkin pie spice
Topping

½ cup (115 g) packed brown sugar

½ cup (4O g) rolled oats

½ teaspoon pumpkin pie spice

Mix pureed banana, pumpkin, sugar, milk, oil, and egg until well blended. Combine flour, baking powder, and pumpkin pie spice. Spoon into muffin pans coated with nonstick vegetable oil spray. Top each with 1 tablespoon of the sugar-spice mixture. Bake in preheated 375°F (190°C, gas mark 5) oven for 20 minutes or until toothpick inserted into muffin comes out clean.

Yield: 12 servings

Each with: 19 g water; 195 calories (26% from fat, 7% from protein, 67% from carb); 4 g protein; 6 g total fat; 1 g saturated fat; 3 g monounsaturated fat; 2 g polyunsaturated fat; 34 g carb; 3 g fiber; 18 g sugar; 112 mg phosphorus; 74 mg calcium; 1 mg iron; 96 mg sodium; 151 mg potassium; 1629 IU vitamin A; 11 mg vitamin E; 0 mg vitamin C; 18 mg cholesterol

15 Blueberry Oatmeal Muffins

Here are some quick muffins with a great blueberry taste.

C cups (C84 g) biscuit baking mix

½ cup (115 g) packed brown sugar

¾ cup (6O g) quick-cooking oats 1 teaspoon cinnamon

2 eggs, well beaten

1½ cups (C55 ml) skim milk

¼ cup (55 g) unsalted butter, melted2 cups (29O g) blueberries

Combine biscuit mix, brown sugar, oats, and cinnamon. Mix eggs, milk, and butter. Add dry ingredients all at once and stir until just blended; fold in blueberries. Spoon into muffin pans coated with nonstick vegetable oil spray, filling each cup two-thirds full. Bake in preheated 400°F (200°C, gas mark 6) oven for 15 to 20 minutes. Remove from pans and place on rack to cool.

Yield: 18 servings

Each with: 40 g water; 167 calories (34% from fat, 9% from protein, 57% from carb); 4 g protein; 6 g total fat; 3 g saturated fat; 3 g monounsaturated fat; 1 g polyunsaturated fat; 24 g carb; 2 g fiber; 10g sugar; 166 mg phosphorus; 77 mg calcium; 1 mg iron; 266 mg sodium; 124 mg potassium; 161 IU vitamin A; 43 mg vitamin E; 2 mg vitamin C; 34 mg cholesterol

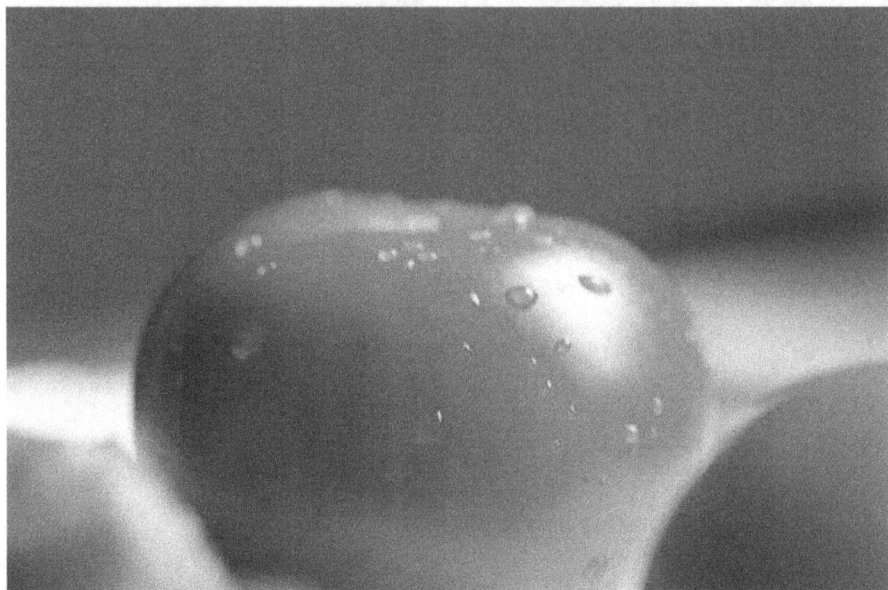

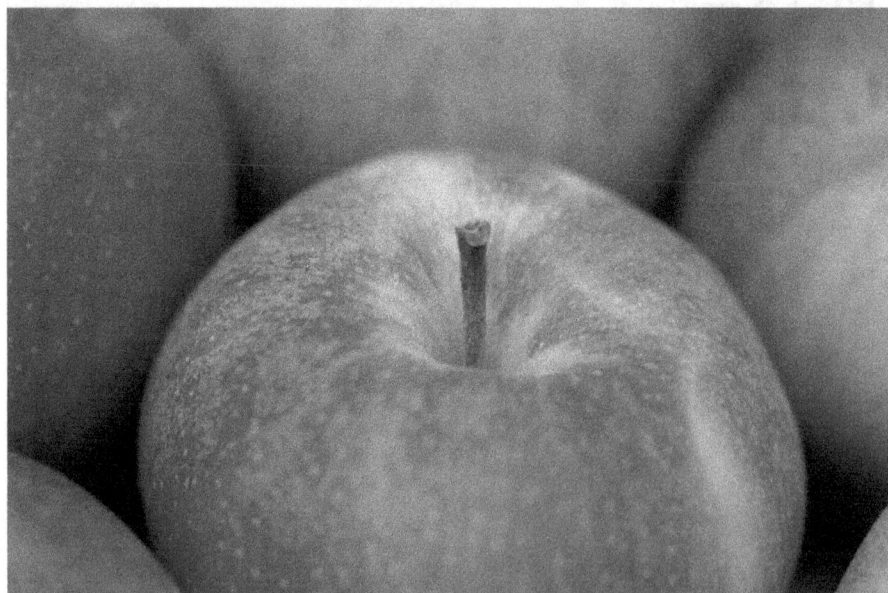

Main Dishes

Moving into main dishes, we start with legumes. You probably think of chili immediately. And we have some chili recipes, but we also have a variety of other soups, casseroles, and main-dish salads containing a wide variety of different kinds of beans.

16 Old-Fashioned Vegetable Soup

This is a summer vegetable soup full of good things from the garden.

2 cups (48O g) no-salt-added canned tomatoes 1 quart (946 ml) low-sodium chicken broth

½ cup (8O g) chopped onion

½ cup (5O g) chopped celery2 bay leaves

2 ½ teaspoons basil, divided

½ teaspoon black pepper

2 cups (14O g) coarsely chopped cabbage

½ cup (5O g) cauliflower1 teaspoon parsley flakes 1 cup corn

1 cup (1CO g) sliced carrot

1 cup (11C g) sliced zucchini2 potatoes, peeled and diced

Place tomatoes in a large pot with broth. Bring to a boil. Add onion and celery, bay leaves, 1½ teaspoons basil, and black pepper. Cover and simmerfor 1 hour.

Add cabbage, cauliflower, parsley, corn, carrot, zucchini, and potato. Cover and simmer until vegetables are tender, 45 to 60 minutes longer. Add remaining basil; simmer 5 minutes longer. Remove bay leaves before serving.

Yield: 8 servings

Each with: 312 g water; 130 calories (8% from fat, 17% from protein, 75% from carb); 6 g protein;

1 g total fat; 0 g saturated fat; 0 g monounsaturated fat; 0 g polyunsaturated fat; 27 g carb; 4 g fiber; 4

g sugar; 138 mg phosphorus; 44 mg calcium; 2 mg iron; 70 mg sodium; 816 mg potassium; 3030 IUvitamin A; 0 mg vitamin E; 35 mg vitamin C; 0 mg cholesterol

17 Pumpkin Soup

This soup can be sipped from a mug or packed in a travel mug and takenwith you.

½ cup (8O g) chopped onion

½ teaspoon minced garlic 1 teaspoon (5 ml) olive oil

½ cup (9O g) chopped tomato 2 cups (49O g) pumpkin

2 cups (475 ml) low-sodium chicken broth

½ teaspoon paprika

1½ teaspoons curry powder

In a large saucepan, cook the onion and garlic in the oil until tender, 2 to 3 minutes. Stir in the remaining ingredients and heat to boiling. Reduce heat, cover, and simmer 10 minutes, stirring occasionally, until vegetables are tender. Place in blender and process until smooth.

Yield: 4 servings

Each with: 261 g water; 86 calories (22% from fat, 18% from protein, 60% from carb); 4 g protein;
2 g total fat; 1 g saturated fat; 1 g monounsaturated fat; 0 g polyunsaturated fat; 15 g carb; 4 g fiber; 6
g sugar; 93 mg phosphorus; 48 mg calcium; 2 mg iron; 44 mg sodium; 449 mg potassium; 19380 IUvitamin A; 0 mg vitamin E; 9 mg vitamin C; 0 mg cholesterol

18 Pumpkin Vegetable Soup

This easy soup has a lot of flavor, both from the vegetables and the curry powder. To make it vegetarian, substitute vegetable broth for the chicken and omit the chicken breast.

½ cup (8O g) chopped onion

½ teaspoon minced garlic 1 teaspoon (5 ml) olive oil 2 cups (C1O g) mixed vegetables, frozen 1 can pumpkin can no-salt-added canned tomatoes

½ cup (12O ml) water 1½ teaspoons curry powder

½ teaspoon paprika

1 cups (475 ml) low-sodium chicken broth

1 cup (14O g) chopped cooked chicken breast

In a large saucepan, cook the onion and garlic in the oil until tender, 2 to 3 minutes. Stir in the remaining ingredients and heat to boiling. Reduce heat, cover, and simmer 10 minutes, stirring occasionally, until vegetables are tender.

Yield: 4 servings

Each with: 261 g water; 158 calories (19% from fat, 42% from protein, 39% from carb); 16 g protein; 3 g total fat; 1 g saturated fat; 2 g monounsaturated fat; 1 g polyunsaturated fat; 15 g carb; 5 g fiber; 4 g sugar; 172 mg phosphorus; 43 mg calcium; 2 mg iron; 442 mg sodium; 396 mg potassium; 4059 IU vitamin A; 2 mg vitamin E; 5 mg vitamin C; 30 mg cholesterol

19 Tomato Vegetable Soup

This recipe starts with a cream of tomato-type soup and then adds to it toend up with a really good spicy vegetable soup.

1 cup (16O g) finely chopped onion

½ teaspoon finely chopped garlic

½ cup (75 g) finely chopped green bell pepper 1 cup (2C5 ml) low-sodium chicken broth
½ cup (115 g) canned corn

½ cup (11C g) canned peas1 cup (1O5 g) macaroni
1 teaspoon low-sodium beef bouillon

2 cups (48O g) no-salt-added canned tomatoes

½ cup (C4 g) nonfat dry milk powder

¼ teaspoon salt-free seasoning blend, such as Mrs. Dash

¼ teaspoon white pepper1½ cups (C55 ml) water
¼ cup (C4 g) jalapeño peppers, roasted and minced

Sauté onion, garlic, and bell pepper until well cooked. Set aside. In a separate pot, combine chicken broth, juice from corn and peas, plus enough water to cook the macaroni (close to a quart). Bring to boil. Add macaroni. Cook for 12 minutes. Drain the macaroni and store broth for next time. Puree the bouillon, tomatoes, dry milk, seasonings, water, and sautéed onion, garlic, and bell pepper. Combined pureed sauce, macaroni, peas, corn, and minced jalapeños and simmer for 30 minutes.

Yield: 4 servings

Each with: 371 g water; 174 calories (6% from fat, 21% from protein, 73% from carb); 10 g protein; 1 g total fat; 0 g saturated fat; 0 g monounsaturated fat; 0 g polyunsaturated fat; 34 g carb; 5 g fiber;

12 g sugar; 196 mg phosphorus; 168 mg calcium; 2 mg iron; 108 mg sodium; 625 mg potassium; 926IU vitamin A; 60 mg vitamin E; 36 mg vitamin C; 2 mg cholesterol

20 Vegetable Pasta Sauce

This pasta sauce can't be beat. It's low in calories, fat free, has 3 grams of fiber, and a great Italian flavor on top of all that.

1 cup (16O g) finely chopped onion 1 teaspoon crushed garlic

2 teaspoons basil

1½ teaspoons oregano1 bay leaf

28 ounces (8OO g) no-salt-added canned tomatoes

16 ounces (455 g) no-salt-added tomato sauce

¼ teaspoon black pepper, fresh ground

4 tablespoons (16 g) chopped fresh parsley

In a large pot, heat onion, garlic, basil, oregano, bay leaf, tomatoes, tomato sauce, pepper, and parsley. Mix well, mashing tomatoes with a fork. Bring to boiling, reduce heat, and simmer uncovered, stirring occasionally, for 1½ hours. Remove bay leaf. Serve over whole wheat pasta.

Yield: 6 servings

Each with: 218 g water; 64 calories (5% from fat, 14% from protein, 81% from carb); 2 g protein; 0 g total fat; 0 g saturated fat; 0 g monounsaturated fat; 0 g polyunsaturated fat; 14 g carb; 3 g fiber; 8 g sugar; 61 mg phosphorus; 71 mg calcium; 2 mg iron; 28 mg sodium; 597 mg potassium; 668 IUvitamin A; 0 mg vitamin E; 28 mg vitamin C; 0 mg cholesterol

21 Beef, Bean, and Cabbage Stew

This is another recipe based on one sent in by a newsletter subscriber. It makes a great meal with cornbread and a salad.

1 pound (455 g) lean ground beef

½ cup (8O g) chopped onion

1 cup (7O g) cole slaw mix or shredded cabbage

2 cups (48O g) canned no-salt-added canned tomatoes2 cups (C42 g) cooked Mexican beans
1 cup (2C5 ml) water

Break beef up into fine pieces and brown with the chopped onion and slaw mix or cabbage until the vegetables become clear. Add tomatoes, beans, and water. Bring to boil and simmer 10 minutes to blend the flavors.

Yield: 5 servings

Ech with: 265 g water; 345 calories (39% from fat, 35% from protein, 25% from carb); 30 g protein; 15 g total fat; 6 g saturated fat; 7 g monounsaturated fat; 1 g polyunsaturated fat; 22 g carb; 8 g fiber; 3 g sugar; 268 mg phosphorus; 95 mg calcium; 5 mg iron; 83 mg sodium; 818 mg potassium; 132 IU vitamin A; 0 mg vitamin E; 18 mg vitamin C; 73 mg cholesterol

22 Mexican Beef Salad

This is a kind of taco salad without the tortillas, this makes a great lightdinner for a hot day.

1 pound (455 g) ground beef, extra lean

½ cup (8O g) chopped onion 1 tablespoon chili powder teaspoons oregano ½ teaspoon cumin

1 cup (1OO g) cooked kidney beans, drained and rinsed 1 pound (455 g) chickpeas, drained and rinsed

1 cup (18O g) diced tomato

2 cups (11O g) iceberg lettuce

½ cup (58 g) shredded Cheddar cheese

Cook ground beef and onion in a skillet over medium-high heat until beef is no longer pink, 10 to 12 minutes. Drain. Stir in chili powder, oregano, and cumin. Cook for 1 minute. Mix in beans, chickpeas, and tomato. Portion lettuce onto serving plates. Top with shredded cheese. Then top with beef mixture.

Yield: 4 servings

Each with: 263 g water; 601 calories (42% from fat, 27% from protein, 31% from carb); 41 gprotein; 28 g total fat; 12 g saturated fat; 11 g monounsaturated fat; 3 g polyunsaturated fat; 47 gcarb; 15 g fiber; 8 g sugar; 525 mg phosphorus; 242 mg calcium; 8 mg iron; 213 mg sodium; 1071 mg potassium; 1284 IU vitamin A; 43 mg vitamin E; 11 mg vitamin C; 96 mg cholesterol

23 Mexican Spaghetti Pie

This is a Mexican-flavored version of spaghetti pie. The kidney beansprovide extra fiber as well as flavor.

12 ounces (C42 g) whole wheat spaghetti 4 tablespoons (55 g) unsalted butter

¼ cup (25 g) grated Parmesan cheese 4 eggs, beaten

½ cup (8O g) chopped onion 1 pound (455 g) ground beef

2 cups (2OO g) cooked kidney beans, drained 2 cups (48O g) no-salt-added canned tomatoes 6 ounces (17O g) no-salt-added tomato paste

4 ounces (115 g) canned green chiles, chopped 2 tablespoons chili powder

1 teaspoon cumin

½ cup (6O g) shredded Monterey Jack cheese

Cook and drain spaghetti and let cool slightly. Stir in butter, Parmesan cheese, and eggs. Spread into the bottom of a large baking dish coated with nonstick vegetable oil spray. Brown onion and ground beef. Stir in kidney beans, undrained tomatoes, and tomato paste. Add chopped green chiles, chili powder, and cumin. Simmer for 30 minutes. Pour meat mixture over pasta in baking dish. Top with the shredded cheese. Bake in a 350°F (180°C, gas mark 4) oven for 30 to 40 minutes or until brown.

Yield: 8 servings

Each with: 152 g water; 607 calories (27% from fat, 25% from protein, 48% from carb); 36 g protein; 17 g total fat; 8 g saturated fat; 5 g monounsaturated fat; 2 g polyunsaturated fat; 68 g carb; 17 g fiber; 6 g sugar; 530 mg phosphorus; 236 mg calcium; 9 mg iron; 232 mg sodium; 1332 mg potassium; 1345 IU vitamin A; 106 mg vitamin E; 14 mg vitamin C; 183 mg cholesterol

24 Southwestern Vegetable Stew

This stew evokes not just the flavor of Mexico, but also that of the southwestern Native American tribes with the use of squash and corn. It's delicious with cornbread.

¾ cup (12O g) chopped onion

½ teaspoon finely chopped garlic 2 tablespoons (28 ml) vegetable oil

1 cup (15O g) red bell pepper, cut into strips

½ cup (72 g) poblano chiles, seeded and cut into strips1 jalapeño pepper, seeded and chopped

1 cup (14O g) cubed acorn squash

4 cups (95O ml) low-sodium chicken broth

½ teaspoon black pepper

½ teaspoon ground coriander

1 cup (11C g) thinly sliced zucchini

1 cup (11C g) thinly sliced yellow squash 1O ounces (28O g) frozen corn

2 cups (C42 g) cooked pinto beans, drained

Cook and stir onion and garlic in oil in 4-quart (4 L) Dutch oven over medium heat until onion is tender. Stir in bell pepper, poblano, and jalapeño. Cook 15 minutes. Stir in squash, broth, black pepper, and coriander. Heat to boiling; reduce heat. Cover and simmer until squash is tender, about 15 minutes. Stir in remaining ingredients. Cook uncovered, stirring occasionally, until zucchini is tender, about 10 minutes.

Yield: 6 servings

Each with: 336 g water; 220 calories (24% from fat, 19% from protein, 57% from carb); 11 g protein; 6 g total fat; 1 g saturated fat; 2 g monounsaturated fat; 3 g polyunsaturated fat; 34 g carb; 8

g fiber; 5 g sugar; 199 mg phosphorus; 58 mg calcium; 2 mg iron; 57 mg sodium; 759 mg potassium; 1001 IU vitamin A; 0 mg vitamin E; 54 mg vitamin C; 0 mg cholesterol

25 Italian Oven Chowder

This Italian dish, halfway between a soup and a casserole, cooks in the oven while you do other things. The cheese and cream make this very rich tasting.

1 cup (11C g) sliced zucchini 1½ cups (24O g) sliced onion cups (C28 g) cooked chickpeas 2 cups (48O g) no-salt-added canned tomatoes, chopped 1½ cups (C55 ml) dry white wine 2 teaspoons minced garlic1 teaspoon basil bay leaf

2 ounces (55 g) shredded Monterey Jack cheese 2 ounces (55 g) grated Romano cheese
1 cup (2C5 ml) whipping cream

Combine zucchini, onion, chickpeas, tomatoes and their liquid, wine, garlic, basil, and bay leaf in 3-quart (3 L) baking dish. Cover and bake at 400°F (200°C, gas mark 6) for 1 hour, stirring once halfway through. Season to taste with salt and pepper. Stir in cheeses and cream. Bake 10 minutes longer. Remove bay leaf before serving. **Yield:** 6 servings

Each with: 258 g water; 309 calories (42% from fat, 16% from protein, 42% from carb); 11 gprotein; 13 g total fat; 7 g saturated fat; 4 g monounsaturated fat; 1 g polyunsaturated fat; 29 g carb; 5g fiber; 5 g sugar; 245 mg phosphorus; 257 mg calcium; 2 mg iron; 427 mg sodium; 485 mgpotassium; 480 IU vitamin A; 81 mg vitamin E; 17 mg vitamin C; 40 mg cholesterol

26 Taco Salad

This recipe is a meal in itself. And you couldn't ask for more flavor.

1 pound (455 g) ground beef 1 tablespoon taco seasoning

2 cups (11O g) shredded lettuce 6 ounces (17O g) corn chips

2 cups (5O4 g) refried beans

1 cup (18O g) chopped tomato

½ cup (8O g) chopped onion

½ cup (75 g) chopped green bell pepper

½ cup (115 g) sour cream

½ cup (1CO g) salsa

Brown the ground beef with the taco seasoning. Drain. Layer lettuce, chips, beef, beans, tomato, onion, and pepper. Top with sour cream and salsa.

Yield: 4 servings

Each with: 318 g water; 523 calories (39% from fat, 25% from protein, 36% from carb); 33 gprotein; 23 g total fat; 10 g saturated fat; 9 g monounsaturated fat; 2 g polyunsaturated fat; 48 g carb; 11 g fiber; 4 g sugar; 438 mg phosphorus; 183 mg calcium; 5 mg iron; 538 mg sodium; 1006 mg potassium; 842 IU vitamin A; 50 mg vitamin E; 31 mg vitamin C; 92 mg cholesterol

27 Texas Cornbread Skillet Meal

This makes a nice meal-in-a-pot sort of dinner. I've also made a meatlessvariation of it for lunch that was every bit as good.

1 pound (455 g) ground beef1 cup (16O g) chopped onion

1 tablespoon minced garlic clove

2 cups (48O g) no-salt-added canned tomatoes 2 cups (C44 g) cooked black-eyed peas, drained 1½ teaspoons Cajun seasoning

½ cup (7O g) cornmeal

½ cup (62 g) flour

1 tablespoon baking powder1 egg

½ cup (12O ml) skim milk

In a large cast-iron or ovenproof skillet, brown ground beef, onion, and garlic. Add undrained tomatoes, black-eyed peas, and seasoning. Stir well. In a separate bowl, combine cornmeal, flour, and baking powder. Stir egg and milk together and then stir into dry ingredients. Top meat mixture with cornbread batter and cook in 425°F (220°C, gas mark 7) oven about 20 to 25 minutes or until cornbread is golden brown.

Yield: 4 servings

Each with: 311 g water; 608 calories (32% from fat, 28% from protein,

39% from carb); 43 g protein; 22 g total fat; 8 g saturated fat; 9 g monounsaturated fat; 2 g polyunsaturated fat; 60 g carb; 9 g fiber; 9 g sugar; 494 mg phosphorus; 334 mg calcium; 8 mg iron; 510 mg sodium; 1086 mg potassium; 394 IU vitamin A; 41 mg vitamin E; 17 mg vitamin C; 145 mg cholesterol

28 Chicken and Black Beans

This is a Mexican-flavored skillet meal featuring marinated chicken andblack beans.

½ cup (12O ml) Italian dressing

½ teaspoon crushed garlic

¼ teaspoon red pepper flakes

12 ounces (C4O g) boneless chicken breast, cut in 1-inch (2.5 cm) cubes2 teaspoons (1O ml) olive oil 1 cup (15O g) chopped green bell pepper

¾ cup (12O g) chopped onion

¾ teaspoon oregano

¼ teaspoon black pepper, fresh ground

¼ teaspoon cumin

2 cups (C44 g) cooked black beans, drained and rinsed 2 cups (48O g) no-salt-added canned tomatoes

¼ cup chopped fresh cilantro

Combine dressing, garlic, and red pepper. Place chicken in large glass bowl, pour dressing over chicken, cover, and refrigerate 30 to 60 minutes (or overnight). Remove chicken from marinade, drain well, and discard marinade. Heat oil in large skillet over medium-high heat until hot. Add chicken, cook 5 to 7 minutes, stirring until chicken is slightly brown, spooning off any excess liquid. Add bell pepper, onion, oregano, pepper, and cumin. Cook, stirring, 4 to 5 minutes or until vegetables are tender. Add black beans and tomatoes. Cook 2 to 3 minutes more or until thoroughly heated. Garnish with cilantro; serve immediately.

Yield: 4 servings

Each with: 314 g water; 355 calories (31% from fat, 32% from protein, 37% from carb); 29 gprotein; 12 g total fat; 2 g saturated fat; 4 g monounsaturated fat; 5 g polyunsaturated fat; 33 g carb;

10 g fiber; 7 g sugar; 332 mg phosphorus; 90 mg calcium; 4 mg iron; 562 mg sodium; 896 mg potassium; 550 IU vitamin A; 5 mg vitamin E; 46 mg vitamin C; 49 mg cholesterol

Side Dishes and Salads

Grains are a natural for side dishes. Rice is probably the one you think of first, but don't ignore other choices such as barley and bulgur. We've included a number of recipes here to get you thinking about them.

29 Potato Dumplings

Try these with sauerbraten or just plain grilled pork chops.

4 potatoes

1 egg, beaten

C tablespoons (24 g) cornstarch

1 cup (115 g) whole wheat bread crumbs

¼ teaspoon black pepper

¼ cup (C1 g) flour

Peel potatoes and boil in salted water until soft. Drain and mash until smooth. Blend in eggs, cornstarch, bread crumbs, and pepper. Mix thoroughly and shape into dumplings. You may need to add flour to make dumplings hold together. Roll each dumpling in flour and drop into rapidly boiling water. Cover and cook for about 15 or 20 minutes.

Yield: 6 servings

Each with: 163 g water; 271 calories (7% from fat, 10% from protein,

83% from carb); 7 g protein;

2 g total fat; 1 g saturated fat; 1 g monounsaturated fat; 1 g polyunsaturated fat; 57 g carb; 4 g fiber; 3

g sugar; 128 mg phosphorus; 54 mg calcium; 2 mg iron; 48 mg sodium; 703 mg potassium; 51 IUvitamin A; 13 mg vitamin E; 15 mg vitamin C; 39 mg cholesterol

30 Potato and Vegetable Hash

Adding vegetables makes hash-browned potatoes a more complete sidedish, but they are still good for breakfast this way too. Depending on the meal, a number of different herbs could be added. We sprinkle them with a little garlic powder and basil just before turning.

2 potatoes, shredded

½ cup (8O g) shredded onion

¼ cup (C8 g) shredded red bell pepper

¼ cup (C8 g) shredded green bell pepper

¼ cup (28 g) shredded zucchini cup (6O g) finely chopped tomato

2 tablespoons (28 ml) olive oil

Shred all vegetables except tomato. Mix together. Heat oil in a large skillet. Add vegetables and spread to an even layer. Cook until lightly browned. Turn over and add chopped tomato on top. Cover and cook until tender. Cutin wedges to serve.

Yield: 6 servings

Each with: 114 g water; 136 calories (30% from fat, 6% from protein, 64% from carb); 2 g protein; 5 g total fat; 1 g saturated fat; 3 g monounsaturated fat; 1 g polyunsaturated fat; 22 g carb; 2 g fiber; 2 g sugar; 51 mg phosphorus; 14 mg calcium; 0 mg iron; 7 mg sodium; 404 mg potassium; 300 IUvitamin A; 0 mg vitamin E; 23 mg vitamin C; 0 mg cholesterol

31 Avocado and Crabmeat Salad

This is another of those "fancy" salads that are good when you have guests. But go ahead and treat yourself even if there is no one but family. This makes enough that it could be a whole meal in itself.

1 cup (2CO g) fat-free sour cream

4 tablespoons (64 g) low-fat mayonnaise1 teaspoon Worcestershire sauce

1 avocado

1 cup asparagus, cut in 1-inch (2.5 cm) pieces

¼ cup (25 g) sliced black olives 1 pound (455 g) crabmeat

1 can artichoke hearts, quartered

Combine sour cream, mayonnaise, and Worcestershire to make sauce. Peel and coarsely chop avocado. Combine asparagus, black olives, crabmeat, artichoke, and avocado. Pour sauce over salad and mix.

Yield: 8 servings

Each with: 130 g water; 172 calories (42% from fat, 38% from protein, 20% from carb); 14 g protein; 7 g total fat; 1 g saturated fat; 2 g monounsaturated fat; 1 g polyunsaturated fat; 7 g carb; 3 g fiber; 1 g sugar; 229 mg phosphorus; 82 mg calcium; 1 mg iron; 740 mg sodium; 396 mg potassium; 361 IU vitamin A; 35 mg vitamin E; 10 mg vitamin C; 44 mg cholesterol

32 Broccoli and Tomato Salad

As pretty as it is tasty, this salad is great with a piece of grilled meat or anegg dish like quiche.

1 pound (455 g) broccoli

¼ pound (115 g) mushrooms

¾ cup (75 g) olives, drained

8 ounces (225 g) cherry tomatoes
Dressing

⅓ cup (80 ml) olive oil

1 tablespoon (15 ml) white wine vinegar 1 tablespoon (15 ml) lemon juice
2 tablespoons chopped fresh parsley

¼ cup (25 g) minced scallions

¼ teaspoon minced garlic

¼ teaspoon black pepper, fresh ground

Trim florets from broccoli, you should have about 1 quart (1 L). Reserve stems for another use. Drop broccoli florets into boiling water for 1 minute or just until they turn bright green; drain. Trim mushroom stems to ½ inch (1 cm). Combine broccoli, mushrooms, olives, and cherry tomatoes in bowl. Measure oil, vinegar, lemon juice, parsley, scallions, garlic, and pepper into small bowl. Whisk until blended. Pour dressing over vegetable mixture. Turn gently to coat vegetables. Cover and refrigerate 3 hours or more until ready to serve.

Yield: 4 servings

Each with: 162 g water; 249 calories (72% from fat, 7% from protein, 20% from carb); 5 g protein; 21 g total fat; 3 g saturated fat; 15 g monounsaturated fat; 2 g polyunsaturated fat; 13 g carb; 5 gfiber; 3 g sugar; 104 mg phosphorus; 88 mg calcium; 2 mg iron; 261 mg sodium; 603 mg potassium; 1351 IU vitamin A; 0 mg vitamin E; 117 mg vitamin C; 0 mg cholesterol

33 Broccoli Cauliflower Salad

This simple salad is good with grilled meat or any of a number of othermeals.

1 pound (455 g) broccoli, cut in florets

1 pound (455 g) cauliflower, cut in florets 1 cup (16O g) thinly sliced red onion

½ cup (115 g) mayonnaise

¼ cup (6O ml) vinegar

¼ cup (5O g) sugar

¼ cup (6O ml) salad oil

C tablespoons (45 ml) mustard

Mix broccoli and cauliflower florets. Add onion and combine otheringredients. Pour over vegetables. Refrigerate 2 hours before serving.

Yield: 6 servings

Each with: 174 g water; 307 calories (69% from fat, 6% from protein, 25% from carb); 4 g protein; 24 g total fat; 4 g saturated fat; 10 g monounsaturated fat; 9 g polyunsaturated fat; 20 g carb; 4 gfiber; 13 g sugar; 88 mg phosphorus; 63 mg calcium; 1 mg iron; 143 mg sodium; 413 mg potassium; 538 IU vitamin A; 15 mg vitamin E; 103 mg vitamin C; 7 mg cholesterol

34 Cabbage Fruit Salad

This is a great dish for fall when cabbage and apples are in season. It features a sweet creamy dressing.

2 cups (14O g) raw, shredded cabbage 1 medium apple, diced and unpeeled 1 tablespoon (15 ml) lemon juice

½ cup (75 g) raisins

¼ cup (6O ml) pineapple juice 1 ½ teaspoons lemon juice

1 tablespoon sugar

½ cup (115 g) sour cream

Prepare cabbage and apple. Use lemon juice to wet apple to prevent darkening. Toss cabbage, raisins, and apple. Mix fruit juices and sugar. Add sour cream and stir until smooth; add to salad and chill.

Yield: 4 servings

Each with: 102 g water; 169 calories (31% from fat, 5% from protein, 64% from carb); 2 g protein; 6 g total fat; 4 g saturated fat; 2 g monounsaturated fat; 0 g polyunsaturated fat; 29 g carb; 2 g fiber; 20 g sugar; 58 mg phosphorus; 64 mg calcium; 1 mg iron; 24 mg sodium; 338 mg potassium; 244 IU vitamin A; 50 mg vitamin E; 24 mg vitamin C; 13 mg cholesterol

35 Corn Salad

Because it is slightly sweet from the apple and very crunchy, this salad isgreat with barbecued meats.

1 cup (15O g) diced green bell pepper 1 avocado, cubed

1 cup (15O g) chopped apple

2 cups (C28 g) corn, cooked and cooled 1 teaspoon Dijon mustard

1 tablespoon (15 ml) red wine vinegar C tablespoons (45 ml) olive oil

Place pepper, avocado, apple, and corn in salad bowl. Stir to mix. Combineremaining ingredients and pour over salad, tossing lightly.

Yield: 4 servings

Each with: 151 g water; 234 calories (56% from fat, 5% from protein, 38% from carb); 3 g protein; 16 g total fat; 2 g saturated fat; 11 g monounsaturated fat; 2 g polyunsaturated fat; 24 g carb; 5 gfiber; 6 g sugar; 77 mg phosphorus; 14 mg calcium; 1 mg iron; 23 mg sodium; 386 mg potassium; 201 IU vitamin A; 0 mg vitamin E; 37 mg vitamin C; 0 mg cholesterol

36 Date Apple Waldorf Salad

Here's another fruity, sweet dessert or salad. This is the kind of thing that kids love (and older people too).

1 orange

2 cups (COO g) diced unpeeled apple

½ cup (75 g) dates, snipped

½ cup (5O g) chopped celery cup (4O g) chopped walnuts

¼ cup (6O g) mayonnaise 1 tablespoon sugar

¾ cup (56 g) whipped dessert topping (such as Cool Whip), thawed

Peel orange; section over bowl to catch juices. Halve sections and reserve 1 tablespoon juice. In medium bowl, combine apple, dates, celery, walnuts, and orange sections. Blend together mayonnaise, sugar, and reserved orange juice. Fold in the whipped dessert topping; combine with date mixture.

Yield: 6 servings

Each with: 76 g water; 211 calories (53% from fat, 5% from protein, 42% from carb); 3 g protein; 13 g total fat; 2 g saturated fat; 3 g monounsaturated fat; 6 g polyunsaturated fat; 24 g carb; 3 g fiber; 19g sugar; 64 mg phosphorus; 37 mg calcium; 0 mg iron; 69 mg sodium; 258 mg potassium; 202 IU vitamin A; 21 mg vitamin E; 18 mg vitamin C; 9 mg cholesterol

37 Fiesta Salad

This simple but flavorful main-dish salad is good for those warmer springevenings.

2 tablespoons (28 ml) olive oil

2 tablespoons (28 ml) lime juice

1 tablespoon (15 ml) lemon juice

¼ teaspoon garlic powder

½ teaspoon cumin

¼ teaspoon oregano

1 boneless chicken breast

4 cups (22O g) romaine lettuce16 cherry tomatoes 1 avocado, peeled and sliced

¼ cup (27 g) shredded Swiss cheese

½ cup (C6 g) crumbled tortilla chips

2 tablespoons (CO g) fat-free sour cream

¼ cup (65 g) salsa

Combine first 6 ingredients in a resealable plastic bag. Add chicken breast and marinate at least 2 hours, turning occasionally. Grill or sauté chicken breast until no longer pink. Cut into ½-inch-thick (1 cm) slices. Divide lettuce between two plates. Top with tomatoes, avocado, and chicken. Sprinkle with cheese and tortilla chips. Combine sour cream and salsa and pour over salad.

Yield: 2 servings

Each with: 236 g water; 457 calories (55% from fat, 16% from protein, 28% from carb); 19 g protein; 28 g total fat; 4 g saturated fat; 18 g monounsaturated fat; 4 g polyunsaturated fat; 32 g carb; 10 g fiber; 3 g sugar; 315 mg phosphorus; 268 mg calcium; 3 mg iron; 263 mg sodium; 1187 mg potassium; 6614 IU vitamin A; 24 mg vitamin E; 64 mg vitamin C; 33 mg cholesterol

38 Grapefruit, Avocado, and Spinach Salad

This is a great salad. I like to make a double batch of the dressing and use half to marinate boneless chicken breasts to grill as an accompaniment.

1½ pounds (68O g) fresh spinachC red grapefruit
2 avocados

¼ cup (6O ml) orange juice

2 tablespoons (CO ml) lemon juice1 teaspoon sugar
2 tablespoons (28 ml) white wine vinegar

½ cup (12O ml) olive oil

Remove stems from spinach. Wash spinach thoroughly and dry. Tear leaves into bite-size pieces. Wrap gently in paper towels and refrigerate in plastic bags until ready to toss salad. Peel and section grapefruit. Slice avocados into quarters and then cut each slice into 2-inch (5 cm) chunks. Combine remaining ingredients for dressing. At serving time, toss spinach with dressing. Add grapefruit and avocados and gently toss again. Or arrange grapefruit and avocado slices on bed of dressed spinach on individual serving plates. Pass additional dressing, if desired.

Yield: 6 servings

Each with: 240 g water; 422 calories (52% from fat, 7% from protein,

41% from carb); 8 g protein; 26 g total fat; 4 g saturated fat; 18 g monounsaturated fat; 3 g polyunsaturated fat; 45 g carb; 10 gfiber; 2 g sugar; 138 mg phosphorus; 43 mg calcium; 2 mg iron; 8 mg sodium; 465 mg potassium; 397 IU vitamin A; 0 mg vitamin E; 55 mg vitamin C; 0 mg cholesterol

39 Orange Avocado Salad

Fresh and citrusy with a sesame/poppyseed dressing, this salad would dress up any meal. It's particularly good with chicken or fish.

2 tablespoons (4O g) honey 1 tablespoon sesame seeds1 teaspoon poppyseeds

2 tablespoons (28 ml) vegetable oil

2 tablespoons (28 ml) cider vinegar

¼ teaspoon Worcestershire sauce

¼ teaspoon onion powder

4 cups (22O g) lettuce, torn into bite-size pieces 2 oranges, separated into sections

1 avocado, diced

Combine first 4 ingredients in blender until well blended. With blender running, add oil, vinegar, and Worcestershire sauce in a slow, steady stream. Blend until thickened. Toss lettuce, oranges, and avocado. Drizzle with dressing.

Yield: 4 servings

Each with: 183 g water; 209 calories (51% from fat, 4% from protein, 45% from carb); 2 g protein; 13 g total fat; 2 g saturated fat; 5 g monounsaturated fat; 5 g polyunsaturated fat; 25 g carb; 5 g fiber; 19 g sugar; 54 mg phosphorus; 67 mg calcium; 1 mg iron; 14 mg sodium; 461 mg potassium; 621 IU vitamin A; 0 mg vitamin E; 55 mg vitamin C; 0 mg cholesterol

40 Spnach and Orange Section Salad

A great salad, this could easily be made a full meal by adding some chickenor shrimp.

1 pound (455 g) spinach, washed, trimmed, and drained

½ pound (C5 g) sliced cleaned mushrooms

**5 ounces (14O g) water chestnuts, drained and rinsed4 oranges, peeled and sectioned
2 tablespoons (28 ml) orange juice**

1 tablespoon (15 ml) soy sauce

¼ teaspoon dry mustard

⅛aspoon black pepper, fresh ground

Tear spinach into bite-size pieces. Toss with mushrooms, water chestnuts, and orange sections. Combine remaining ingredients in a jar with a tight-fitting lid. Shake well. Before serving, pour over spinach mixture; toss lightly.

Yield: 8 servings

Each with: 174 g water; 88 calories (5% from fat, 18% from protein, 78% from carb); 4 g protein; 1 g total fat; 0 g saturated fat; 0 g monounsaturated fat; 0 g polyunsaturated fat; 19 g carb; 5 g fiber; 10g sugar; 79 mg phosphorus; 127 mg calcium; 1 mg iron; 125 mg sodium; 543 mg potassium; 7049 IU vitamin A; 0 mg vitamin E; 53 mg vitamin C; 0 mg cholesterol

Breads

Whole grain breads and rolls are a great way to add extra fiber to your diet. We have a number of yeast bread recipes here that will help you do just that. But don't stop there; we also have recipes for whole grain biscuits and cornbread and for making your own higher-fiber tortillas, flatbread, pizza crust, and bagels.

41 Multigrain Rolls

This makes a nice crunchy, chewy sort of roll, perfect for mild-flavored fillings like turkey or egg salad.

1¼ (295 ml) cups water

C tablespoons nonfat dry milk powder 1½ tablespoons (25 ml) oil

C tablespoons (6O g) molasses 2½ cups (C42 g) bread flour 1 cup 7-grain cereal

2 teaspoons yeast

C tablespoons (24 g) sesame seeds

Place all ingredients in bread machine in order specified by manufacturer. Process on dough cycle. Remove from bread machine at the end of cycle, form into rolls, cover, and let rise until doubled. Bake at 375°F (190°C, gas mark 5) until golden brown, about 15 minutes.

Yield: 10 servings

Each with: 37 g water; 212 calories (18% from fat, 12% from protein, 70% from carb); 7 g protein;
4 g total fat; 1 g saturated fat; 1 g monounsaturated fat; 2 g polyunsaturated fat; 38 g carb; 3 g fiber; 4
g sugar; 119 mg phosphorus; 68 mg calcium; 3 mg iron; 12 mg sodium; 239 mg potassium; 31 IU vitamin A; 9 mg vitamin E; 0 mg vitamin C; 0 mg cholesterol

42 Rye Rolls

This is another good sandwich roll. I like my roast beef on rye, personally.

1 cup (2C5 ml) skim milk

1½ tablespoons (21 g) unsalted butter1 egg
1½ cups (2O5 g) bread flour2 cups (256 g) rye flour
¼ cup (5O g) sugar

1 tablespoon caraway seed 2 tablespoons (24 g) yeast

Place all ingredients in bread machine in order specified by manufacturer. Process on dough cycle. At end of cycle, remove to a floured board. Pull into 10 pieces. Shape each into a rounded, flattened roll and place on baking sheet coated with nonstick vegetable oil spray. Cover and let rise until double, about 30 minutes. Bake in preheated 375°F (190°C, gas mark 5) oven 12 to 15 minutes or until golden brown.

Yield: 10 servings

Each with: 30 g water; 212 calories (14% from fat, 13% from protein, 73% from carb); 7 g protein;
3 g total fat; 1 g saturated fat; 1 g monounsaturated fat; 0 g polyunsaturated fat; 39 g carb; 4 g fiber; 5
g sugar; 132 mg phosphorus; 52 mg calcium; 2 mg iron; 26 mg sodium; 177 mg potassium; 139 IU vitamin A; 38 mg vitamin E; 0 mg vitamin C; 26 mg cholesterol

43 Focaccia Rolls

cup (18O ml) water

2 tablespoons (28 ml) olive oil

2 cups (274 g) bread flour

1 tablespoon sugar

1½ tablespoons (16 g) yeast1 tablespoon basil
1 teaspoon rosemary

2 tablespoons grated Parmesan cheese

Place first 5 ingredients in bread machine in order specified by manufacturer. Process on dough cycle. Remove the dough from machine when cycle ends. Pat into 8 × 12-inch (20 × 30 cm) rectangle on a floured board. Cut into six 4-inch (10 cm) squares. Place on baking sheet sprayed with nonstick vegetable oil spray. Cover and let rise until doubled, about 30 minutes. Make depressions in top at 1-inch (2.5 cm) intervals with finger. Sprinkle herbs and cheese over top. Bake at 400°F (200°C, gas mark 6)until done, 15 to 18 minutes. **Yield:** 6 servings

Each with: 36 g water; 230 calories (23% from fat, 13% from protein, 64% from carb); 7 g protein;
6 g total fat; 1 g saturated fat; 4 g monounsaturated fat; 1 g polyunsaturated fat; 37 g carb; 2 g fiber; 2
g sugar; 97 mg phosphorus; 38 mg calcium; 3 mg iron; 32 mg sodium; 120 mg potassium; 47 IU vitamin A; 2 mg vitamin E; 0 mg vitamin C; 1 mg cholesterol

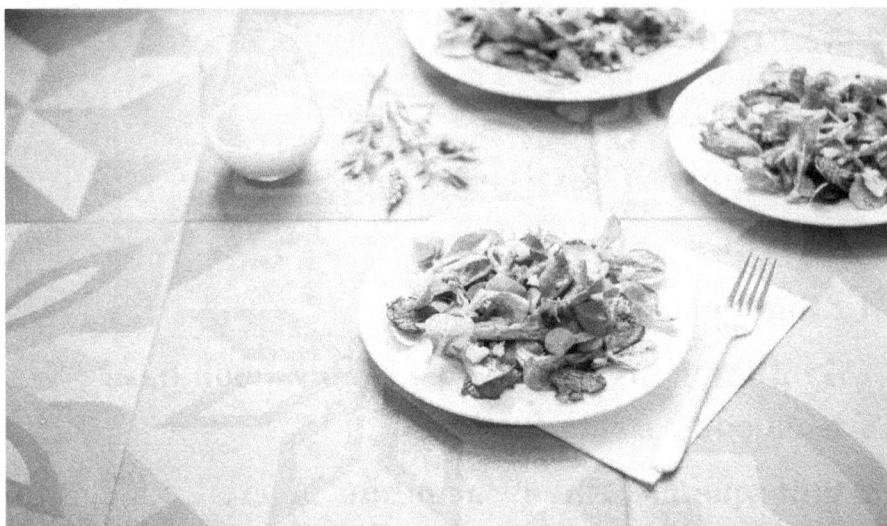

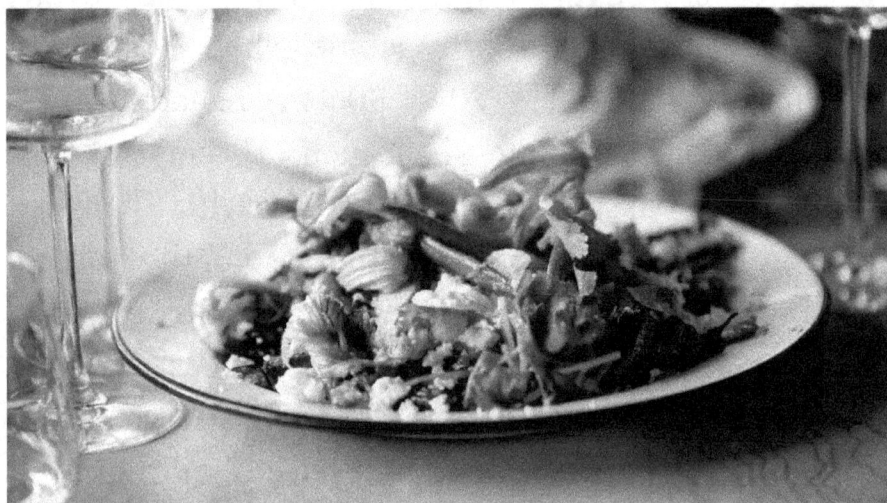

Desserts and Other Sweets

Yes, there actually are recipes for desserts made with legumes. Admittedly there aren't a lot, and a lot of them tend to be kind of similar, but I was so impressed with the whole idea that I decided to go ahead and make it a separate chapter, even if it does only contain two recipes. You really should try the bean pie—it will not be what you expect.

44 Crunchy Orange Cookies

This is a different kind of oatmeal cookie, with a nice, unexpected orange flavor.

1 cup (225 g) unsalted butter 1 cup (2OO g) sugar
2 eggs

¼ cup (6O ml) orange juice 1 teaspoon vanilla extract
2 teaspoons grated orange peel

2 cups (24O g) whole wheat pastry flour 1 teaspoon baking soda
2 cups (16O g) quick-cooking oats 1 cup (145 g) raisins
½ cup (55 g) chopped pecans

Cream butter and sugar until light. Beat in eggs, juice, vanilla, and orange peel. Add dry ingredients and mix well. Stir in oats, raisins, and pecans by hand. Drop by rounded teaspoons on baking sheet coated with nonstick vegetable oil spray. Bake at 375°F (190°C, gas mark 5) for 10 to 15 minutes. Transfer to racks to cool. Store in an airtight container.

Yield: 42 servings

Each with: 6 g water; 117 calories (44% from fat, 7% from protein, 49% from carb); 2 g protein; 6 g total fat; 3 g saturated fat; 2 g monounsaturated fat; 1 g polyunsaturated fat; 15 g carb; 1 g fiber; 7 g sugar; 52 mg phosphorus; 10 mg calcium; 1 mg iron; 5 mg sodium; 80 mg potassium; 151 IU vitamin A; 40 mg vitamin E; 1 mg vitamin C; 23 mg cholesterol

45 Fruit Cookies

Pick your favorite fruit or fruits to make these cookies your own. My personal favorites are cranberries, cherries, and pineapple.

1½ cups (CC7 g) mashed banana cup (8O ml) canola oil 1 teaspoon vanilla extract 1½ cups (12O g) rolled oats ½ cup (5O g) oat bran

1½ cups (24O g) mixed dried fruits, coarsely chopped ½ cup (6O g) chopped walnuts

Preheat oven to 350°F (180°C, gas mark 4). Coat 2 baking sheets with nonstick vegetable oil spray. Mash bananas in a large bowl until smooth. Stir in oil and vanilla. Add oats, oat bran, mixed fruits, and walnuts. Stir well to combine. Drop by rounded teaspoons on baking sheets about 1 inch (2.5 cm) apart. Flatten slightly with back of a spoon. Bake 20 to 25 minutes or until bottom and edges are lightly brown. Cool completely; refrigerate.

Yield: 24 servings

Each with: 23 g water; 115 calories (38% from fat, 6% from protein, 56% from carb); 2 g protein; 5 g total fat; 0 g saturated fat; 2 g monounsaturated fat; 2 g polyunsaturated fat; 17 g carb; 2 g fiber; 9 g sugar; 49 mg phosphorus; 8 mg calcium; 1 mg iron; 4 mg sodium; 139 mg potassium; 28 IU vitamin A; 3 mg vitamin E; 3 mg vitamin C; 0 mg cholesterol

46 Graham Cracker Praline Cookies

These are an easy sort of toffee cookie.

24 graham crackers

1 cup (225 g) unsalted butter

1 cup (225 g) packed dark brown sugar1 cup (11O g) chopped pecans

Place crackers on ungreased baking sheet with an edge. Melt butter and sugar. Bring to a boil. Add pecans and boil 2 minutes, no longer. Pour over graham crackers and bake in 275°F (140°C, gas mark 1) oven for 10minutes. Remove, let cool slightly, and cut into fingers while still warm.

Yield: 48 servings

Each with: 1 g water; 86 calories (61% from fat, 3% from protein, 37% from carb); 1 g protein; 6 g total fat; 3 g saturated fat; 2 g monounsaturated fat; 1 g polyunsaturated fat; 8 g carb; 1 g fiber; 6 g sugar; 12 mg phosphorus; 4 mg calcium; 0 mg iron; 29 mg sodium; 17 mg potassium; 120 IUvitamin A; 32 mg vitamin E; 0 mg vitamin C; 10 mg cholesterol

47 Granola Cookies

These make tasty treats for breakfast or a snack, and they are healthybesides.

1 cup (145 g) firmly packed dates

1 cup (26O g) apple juice concentrateC tablespoons (48 g) peanut butter C tablespoons (6O g) honey 1 teaspoon vanilla extract 1 tablespoon (2O g) molasses tablespoon chopped walnuts

½ cup (4O g) coconut ½ cup (75 g) raisins

1 cups (28O g) whole wheat flour2 cups (16O g) quick-cooking oats

Blend dates and apple juice until smooth. Add peanut butter, honey, vanilla, and molasses. Blend well and place in mixing bowl. Add nuts, coconut, raisins, and flour and mix well. Add oats and blend. Spoon onto nonstick baking sheet; press with wet fork until ¼ inch (0.5 cm) thick. Bake at 300°F (150°C, gas mark 2) about 20 minutes. Cool completely on racks and store in airtight container.

Yield: 36 servings

Each with: 5 g water; 91 calories (15% from fat, 10% from protein, 75% from carb); 2 g protein; 2 g total fat; 0 g saturated fat; 0 g monounsaturated fat; 0 g polyunsaturated fat; 18 g carb; 2 g fiber; 8 g sugar; 61 mg phosphorus; 11 mg calcium; 1 mg iron; 9 mg sodium; 135 mg potassium; 1 IU vitaminA; 0 mg vitamin E; 3 mg vitamin C; 0 mg cholesterol

48 Raisin-Granola Cookies

These are good-tasting snacks that you can feel good about.

1¾ (145 g) cups granola

1½ cups (18O g) whole wheat pastry flour 1 cup (225 g) unsalted butter, softened

¾ cup (15O g) sugar

¾ cup (17O g) packed dark brown sugar1 teaspoon baking soda

1 teaspoon vanilla extract1 egg

1½ cups (22O g) raisins

Preheat oven to 375°F (190°C, gas mark 5). Coat baking sheets with nonstick vegetable oil spray. Into large bowl measure all ingredients except raisins. With mixer at low speed, beat ingredients just until mixed. Increase speed to medium and beat 2 minutes, occasionally scraping bowl withrubber spatula. Stir in raisins until mixture is well blended. Drop dough by heaping teaspoons about 2 inches (5 cm) apart on baking sheets. Bake 12 to 15 minutes until cookies are lightly browned around edges. Remove to wire racks and allow to cool. Store cookies in a tightly covered container up to 1 week.

Yield: 48 servings

Each with: 3 g water; 97 calories (39% from fat, 4% from protein, 57%

from carb); 1 g protein; 4 g total fat; 3 g saturated fat; 1 g monounsaturated fat; 0 g polyunsaturated fat; 14 g carb; 1 g fiber; 9 g sugar; 29 mg phosphorus; 6 mg calcium; 0 mg iron; 19 mg sodium; 53 mg potassium; 126 IUvitamin A; 34 mg vitamin E; 0 mg vitamin C; 15 mg cholesterol

49 Pecan Cookies

Full of pecans and other good things, these are another cookie that you can eat with a little less guilt than usual.

1 cup (11O g) chopped pecans

½ cup (4O g) coconut

¼ cup (C6 g) sesame seeds

½ cup (112 g) unsalted butter

½ cup (1OO g) sugar1 egg
1 teaspoon vanilla extract

¼ cup (6O ml) skim milk

1 cup (12O g) whole wheat pastry flour

½ teaspoon baking soda1 cup (82 g) granola
½ cup (75 g) raisins

Combine pecans, coconut, and sesame seeds on baking sheet, and heat at 350°F (180°C, gas mark 4) until lightly toasted. Cream butter and sugar. Beat in egg, vanilla, and milk. Sift together flour and baking soda. Stir into egg mixture until blended. Stir in granola, pecan mixture, and raisins. Drop by spoonfuls onto baking sheets coated with nonstick vegetable oil spray. Bake at 375°F (190°C, gas mark 5) for 15 to 20 minutes until lightly browned.

Yield: 36 servings

Each with: 4 g water; 95 calories (54% from fat, 6% from protein, 40% from carb); 1 g protein; 6 g total fat; 2 g saturated fat; 2 g monounsaturated fat; 1 g polyunsaturated fat; 10 g carb; 1 g fiber; 5 g sugar; 41 mg phosphorus; 19 mg calcium; 0 mg iron; 13 mg sodium; 64 mg potassium; 94 IU vitamin A; 25 mg vitamin E; 0 mg vitamin C; 13 mg cholesterol

50 Peanut-Granola Cookies

These make a nice, soft, chewy cookie with a great granola flavor.

1¾ cups (145 g) granola 1½ cups (18O g) whole wheat pastry flour 1 cup (225 g) unsalted butter, softened ¾ cup (15O g) sugar ¾ cup (17O g) packed dark brown sugar1 teaspoon baking soda

1 teaspoon vanilla extract1 egg

1 cup (145 g) peanuts, unsalted and coarsely chopped

Preheat oven to 375°F (190°C, gas mark 5). Coat baking sheets with nonstick vegetable oil spray. Measure all ingredients into a large bowl except peanuts. With mixer at low speed, beat ingredients just until mixed. Increase speed to medium and beat 2 minutes. Stir in peanuts until well blended. Drop dough by heaping teaspoons, about 2 inches (5 cm) apart. Bake 12 to 15 minutes until lightly browned around edges. Remove to rack and cool completely. Store in container with tight lid. **Yield:** 48 servings

Each with: 3 g water; 97 calories (39% from fat, 4% from protein, 57% from carb); 1 g protein; 4 g total fat; 3 g saturated fat; 1 g monounsaturated fat; 0 g polyunsaturated fat; 14 g carb; 1 g fiber; 9 g sugar; 29 mg phosphorus; 6 mg calcium; 0 mg iron; 19 mg sodium; 53 mg potassium; 126 IUvitamin A; 34 mg vitamin E; 0 mg vitamin C; 15 mg cholesterol

Heart Healthy Cookbook for Beginners

Wholesome and Tasty Recipes to Prevent Diseases, Lower Cholesterol and Lower Blood Sugar

Julieth Kern

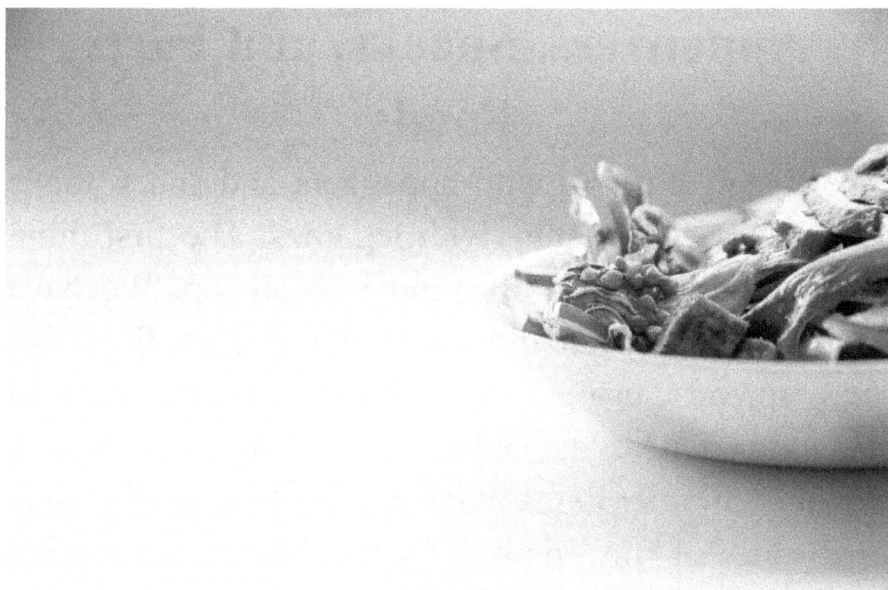

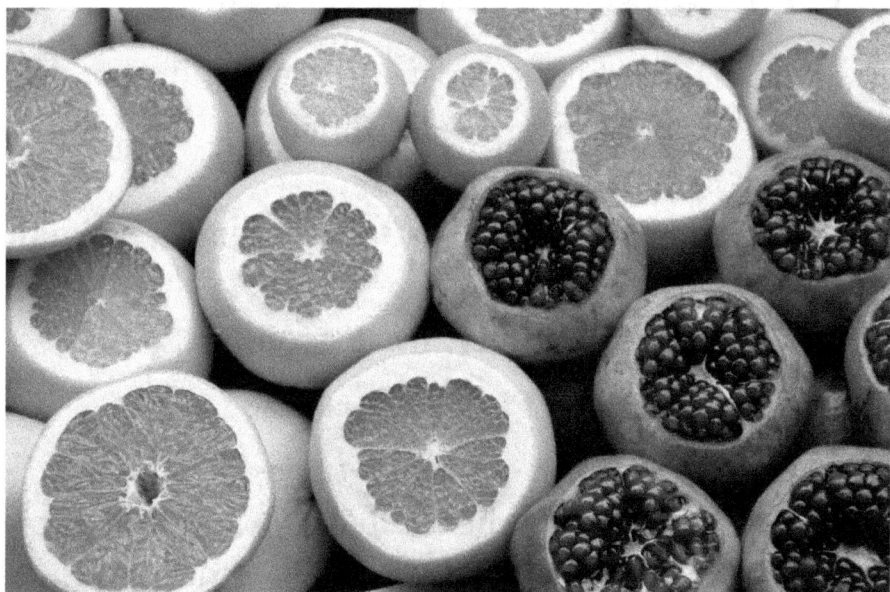

Appetizers, Snacks, and Party Foods

We'll start our trip with appetizers and snack foods and begin that journey with legumes. The first thing that probably comes to mind is bean dip. We have five different bean dips, and you'll also find dips and spreads using less common legumes such as black-eyed peas and chick peas. There are also a number of other items like salsa, nachos, stuffed eggs and one of my new personal favorites, roasted chickpeas.

1 Parmesan-Garlic Pita Toasts

Use these flavorful pita crisps for any of the spreads or dips in the book. Or just nibble on them for a healthier-than-usual snack option.

C tablespoons (42 g) unsalted butter 1 teaspoon minced garlic

½ teaspoon black pepper, fresh ground

¼ cup (25 g) grated Parmesan cheese

2 whole wheat pitas, cut into 8 triangles each

Melt butter; cook garlic in butter over low heat, stirring occasionally, for 5 minutes. Brush mixture lightly on rough side of pita triangles. Arrange butter side up in 1 layer on baking sheet. Sprinkle pepper and Parmesan cheese on top. Bake in oven preheated to 350°F (180°C, gas mark 4) for 12 to 15 minutes, until crisp and light brown. Cool on racks and store inairtight container in a dry place.

Yield: 8 servings

Each with: 7 g water; 95 calories (51% from fat, 12% from protein, 37% from carb); 3 g protein; 6 g total fat; 3 g saturated fat; 1 g monounsaturated fat; 0 g polyunsaturated fat; 9 g carb; 1 g fiber; 0 g sugar; 54 mg phosphorus; 40 mg calcium; 1 mg iron; 134 mg sodium; 35 mg potassium; 147 IU vitamin A; 39 mg vitamin E; 0 mg vitamin C; 14 mg cholesterol

2 Spicy Pita Dippers

Pepper and cumin give these pita triangles a southwestern flavor that goes particularly well with bean dips.

½ cup (112 g) unsalted butter, melted 2 teaspoons lemon pepper

2 teaspoons ground cumin

6 whole wheat pitas, cut into triangles

To make dippers, preheat the broiler. Combine the melted butter, lemon pepper, and cumin in a bowl. Dip the pita pieces quickly in the mixture and then place on a baking sheet. Broil 2 to 4 minutes, until crisp. Cool on a rack.

Yield: 12 servings

Each with: 12 g water; 155 calories (48% from fat, 8% from protein, 44% from carb); 3 g protein; 9 g total fat; 5 g saturated fat; 2 g monounsaturated fat; 1 g polyunsaturated fat; 18 g carb; 2 g fiber; 0 g sugar; 62 mg phosphorus; 12 mg calcium; 1 mg iron; 172 mg sodium; 67 mg potassium; 242 IU vitamin A; 63 mg vitamin E; 0 mg vitamin C; 20 mg cholesterol

3 Whole Wheat Honey Mustard Pretzels

This was one of those extended work-in-progress things as I tried different combinations to get the taste I wanted. The breakthrough was finding the large hard pretzels in a honey wheat with sesame seeds variety from Harry's Premium Snacks at a gourmet food store not too far away. They are great tasting alone, but they also made a great base for this recipe.

¼ cup (55 g) unsalted butter 2 tablespoons (4O g) honey ¼ cup (6O ml) honey mustard

½ teaspoon onion powder

¼ teaspoon Tabasco sauce

8 ounces (225 g) whole wheat pretzels, broken up
Melt butter in microwave. Stir in honey, honey mustard, and spices. Pour over pretzels and stir to coat evenly. Bake at 300°F (150°C, gas mark 2) for 30 minutes, stirring every 10 minutes. Cool on waxed paper. Store in an airtight container.

Yield: 10 servings

Each with: 8 g water; 137 calories (32% from fat, 7% from protein, 60% from carb); 3 g protein; 5 g total fat; 3 g saturated fat; 1 g monounsaturated fat; 0 g polyunsaturated fat; 22 g carb; 2 g fiber; 4 g sugar; 32 mg phosphorus; 9 mg calcium; 1 mg iron; 83 mg sodium; 110 mg potassium; 236 IUvitamin A; 38 mg vitamin E; 1 mg vitamin C; 12 mg cholesterol

4 Ranch-Style Pretzels

These are flavorful pretzel snacks with the taste of ranch dressing.

12 ounces (C4O g) whole wheat pretzels, broken

1 packet Hidden Valley Ranch or other ranch dressing mix1 cup (2C5 ml) olive oil
1 teaspoon lemon pepper1 teaspoon dill weed
1 teaspoon garlic powder

Mix all ingredients in large bowl and toss to coat. Spread on baking sheet. Don't preheat oven. Bake at 300°F (150°C, gas mark 2) for 20 minutes, 10 minutes on one side and then turn and bake another 10 minutes.

Yield: 24 servings

Each with: 1 g water; 132 calories (61% from fat, 5% from protein, 34% from carb); 2 g protein; 9 g total fat; 1 g saturated fat; 7 g monounsaturated fat; 1 g polyunsaturated fat; 12 g carb; 1 g fiber; 0 g sugar; 19 mg phosphorus; 5 mg calcium; 0 mg iron; 29 mg sodium; 65 mg potassium; 3 IU vitamin A; 0 mg vitamin E; 0 mg vitamin C; 0 mg cholesterol

5 Cajun Party Mix

Because it's a little spicier than some party mixes, this one will definitely let you know that you are eating it.

12 ounces (C4O g) almonds

6 cups (18O g) Crispix or other hexagonal multigrain cereal 1 cup (45 g) goldfish-shaped or other small crackers

¼ cup (55 g) unsalted butter

1 tablespoon (15 ml) Worcestershire sauce

½ teaspoon paprika

½ teaspoon thyme

¼ teaspoon black pepper ¼ teaspoon Tabasco sauce Preheat oven to 250°F (120°C, gas mark ½). In a large shallow roasting pan, combine almonds, cereal, and goldfish crackers. Melt butter and stir in seasonings. Pour over mixture and toss to coat. Bake 1 hour, stirring every 20 minutes. Spread on paper towel to cool. Store in an airtight container.

Yield: 36 servings

Each with: 1 g water; 86 calories (61% from fat, 11% from protein, 28% from carb); 2 g protein; 6 g total fat; 1 g saturated fat; 3 g monounsaturated fat; 1 g polyunsaturated fat; 6 g carb; 1 g fiber; 1 g sugar; 51 mg phosphorus; 22 mg calcium; 2 mg iron; 45 mg sodium; 76 mg potassium; 212 IU vitamin A; 55 mg vitamin E; 2 mg vitamin C; 3 mg cholesterol

6 Curried Snack Mix

This is a savory version of the old favorite Chex mix, with curry powder dominating.

2 cups (6O g) round toasted oat cereal, such as Cheerios2 cups (6O g) square wheat cereal, such as Wheat Chex 2 cups (5O g) square rice cereal, such as Rice Chex 2 cups (9O g) pretzel sticks

1½ cups bite-size shredded wheat cereal 1½ teaspoons onion powder 1 teaspoon garlic powder

½ tablespoon curry powder teaspoon ground celery seeds 1½ tablespoons (22 ml) Worcestershire sauce1 teaspoon Tabasco sauce
Combine first 5 ingredients in large roasting pan. Spray thoroughly with nonstick vegetable oil spray. Combine remaining ingredients. Pour over cereal mixture, tossing to coat. Bake at 250°F (120°C, gas mark ½) for 2 hours, stirring and spraying with butter-flavored nonstick cooking spray every 15 minutes. Cool and store in an airtight container.

Yield: 25 servings

Each with: 1 g water; 48 calories (6% from fat, 10% from protein, 83% from carb); 1 g protein; 0 g total fat; 0 g saturated fat; 0 g monounsaturated fat; 0 g polyunsaturated fat; 11 g carb; 1 g fiber; 1 g sugar; 39 mg phosphorus; 27 mg calcium; 4 mg iron; 79 mg sodium; 68 mg potassium; 117 IUvitamin A; 34 mg vitamin E; 3 mg vitamin C; 0 mg cholesterol

7 S'more Snack Mix

This is a great idea. Everyone likes S'mores, so why not a snack mix that gives you that flavor whenever you want it? And all you have to do is mix itup.

1 cups (8O g) honey grahams cereal, such as Golden Grahams 1 cup (5O g) miniature marshmallows

1 cup (145 g) peanuts

½ cup (87.5 g) chocolate chips

½ cup (75 g) raisins

Combine all ingredients and mix thoroughly.

Yield: 20 servings

Each with: 3 g water; 68 calories (29% from fat, 6% from protein, 65% from carb); 1 g protein; 2 g total fat; 1 g saturated fat; 1 g monounsaturated fat; 0 g polyunsaturated fat; 11 g carb; 1 g fiber; 8 g sugar; 24 mg phosphorus; 12 mg calcium; 1 mg iron; 51 mg sodium; 58 mg potassium; 86 IU vitamin A; 26 mg vitamin E; 1 mg vitamin C; 1 mg cholesterol

8 Caramel Corn

This is an easier version than most for caramel corn, not requiring candy thermometers and all that. But the taste is just as good.

½ cup (112 g) unsalted butter 1 cup (225 g) brown sugar

¼ cup (60 ml) corn syrup

½ teaspoon baking soda

4 quarts (128 g) popped popcorn 2 cups (290 g) peanuts

Cook butter, brown sugar, and syrup 1½ minutes; stir and cook an additional 2 to 3 minutes until at a rolling boil. Take off heat and add soda. Stir well. Pour mixture over popped corn and nuts in grocery sack and shake. Microwave 1 minute and shake; 1 minute and shake; 30 seconds and shake; and 30 seconds and shake. Pour into pan, cool, and eat.

Yield: 18 servings

Each with: 5 g water; 184 calories (52% from fat, 4% from protein, 45% from carb); 2 g protein; 11 g total fat; 4 g saturated fat; 3 g monounsaturated fat; 3 g polyunsaturated fat; 21 g carb; 1 g fiber; 13 g sugar; 38 mg phosphorus; 17 mg calcium; 0 mg iron; 164 mg sodium; 74 mg potassium; 173 IU vitamin A; 42 mg vitamin E; 0 mg vitamin C; 14 mg cholesterol

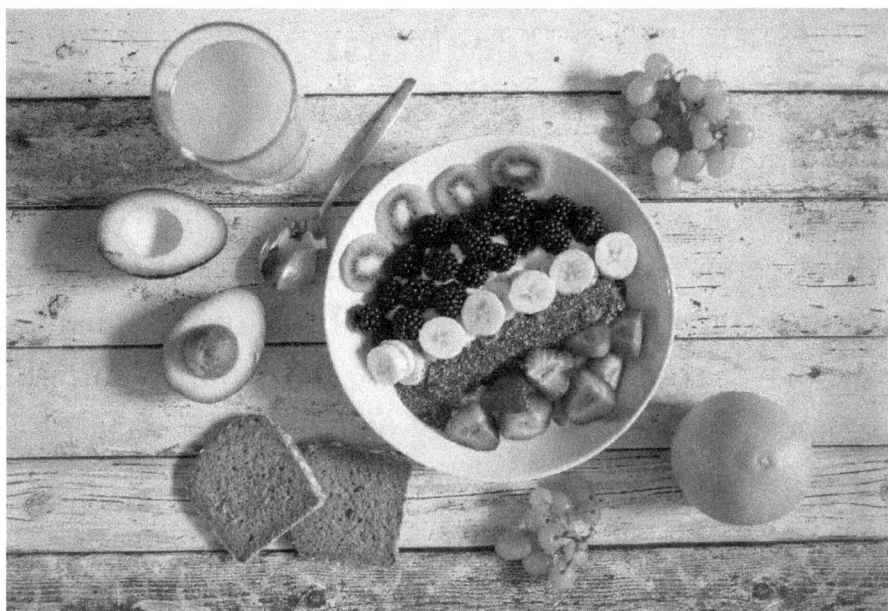

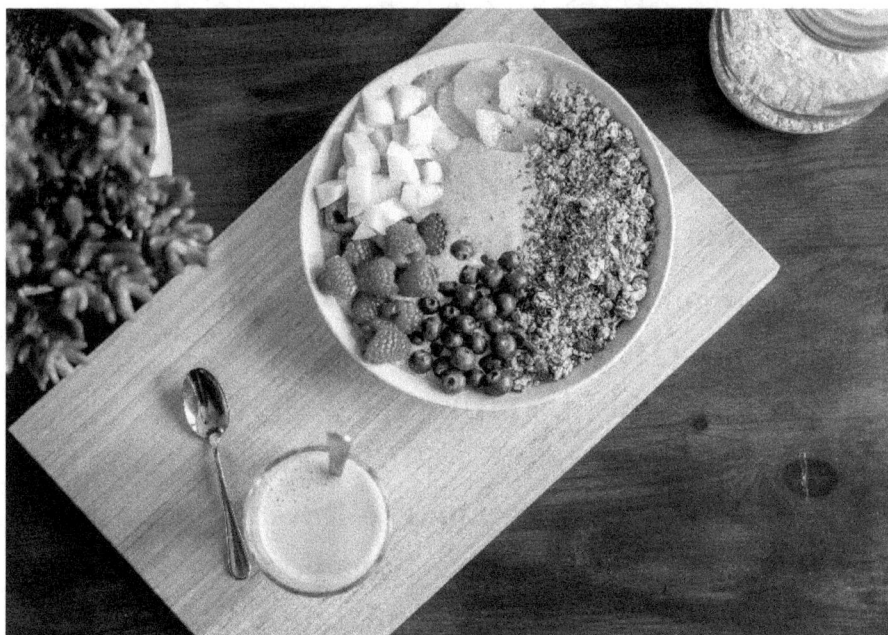

Breakfast

Breakfast is a key meal to get your day started right, and grains are a natural way to do that. Of course, you could choose the quick and easy solution of a high-fiber cereal. But sometimes you want something a little different. At least I know I do. In this chapter we have some ways to spice up your plain old oatmeal, as well as a variety of recipes for pancakes, waffles, scones, and homemade granola.

9 Cinnamon Honey Scones

These are sort of a free-form scone, rather than the more traditional wedges. Serve warm with honey and butter to bring out the flavor of the scones even more.

1¾ cups (220 g) whole wheat pastry flour 1½ teaspoons baking powder

¼ teaspoon cinnamon

6 tablespoons (85 g) unsalted butter, softened 1 tablespoon (20 g) honey

½ cup (120 ml) skim milk 1 egg

Preheat oven to 450°F (230°C, gas mark 8). Line baking sheet with aluminum foil. In a bowl, mix the flour, baking powder, and cinnamon with a wooden spoon. Work butter into mixture by hand until mixture is yellow. Add honey and milk, then egg. Stir with wooden spoon until thoroughly mixed. Scoop spoonful of dough and drop onto baking sheet. Leave 1 inch (2.5 cm) between each. Bake 15 minutes or until golden brown. Cool 5 minutes.

Yield: 8 servings

Each with: 23 g water; 192 calories (45% from fat, 10% from protein, 45% from carb); 5 g protein; 10 g total fat; 6 g saturated fat; 3 g monounsaturated fat; 1 g polyunsaturated fat; 22 g carb; 3 g fiber; 2 g sugar; 142 mg phosphorus; 89 mg calcium; 1 mg iron; 115 mg sodium; 147 mg potassium; 342 IU vitamin A; 92 mg vitamin E; 0 mg vitamin C; 49 mg cholesterol

10 Oatmeal Raisin Scones

I've learned to like scones in recent years. This version not only tastesgreat, but it is healthy too.

2 cups (24O g) whole wheat pastry flour C tablespoons (45 g) brown sugar 1 teaspoon baking powder ½ teaspoon baking soda

½ cup (112 g) unsalted butter, chilled1½ cups (12O g) rolled oats ½ cup (75 g) raisins

1 cup (2C5 ml) buttermilk2 tablespoons cinnamon 2 tablespoons (26 g) sugar

Preheat the oven to 375°F (190°C, gas mark 5). Combine flour, brown sugar, baking powder, and baking soda. Cut in butter until the mixture resembles coarse crumbs. Stir in oats and raisins. Add the buttermilk and mix with a fork until dough forms a ball. Turn out on lightly floured board and knead 6 to 8 minutes. Pat dough into ½-inch (1 cm) thickness. Cut 8 to 10 rounds or wedges and place them on ungreased baking sheet. Sprinkle with sugar and cinnamon. Bake 20 to 25 minutes. **Yield:** 10 servings

Each with: 29 g water; 273 calories (34% from fat, 9% from protein, 57% from carb); 6 g protein; 11 g total fat; 6 g saturated fat; 3 g monounsaturated fat; 1 g polyunsaturated fat; 41 g carb; 5 g fiber; 13 g sugar; 185 mg phosphorus; 97 mg calcium; 2 mg iron; 80 mg sodium; 262 mg potassium; 296 IU vitamin A; 78 mg vitamin E; 1 mg vitamin C; 25 mg cholesterol

11 Whole Grain Scones

The mornings we have these for breakfast, I forgo my usual coffee for a cupof tea.

1 egg

½ cup (100 g) sugar

5 tablespoons (75 ml) canola oil teaspoon lemon peel

½ cup (40 g) rolled oats

¼ cup (25 g) wheat bran

1½ cups (180 g) whole wheat pastry flour 2 tablespoons poppyseeds

1 tablespoon baking powder

½ teaspoon cinnamon

½ cup (120 ml) skim milk
Lemon Topping

C tablespoons (45 ml) lemon juice

¼ cup (25 g) confectioners' sugar

Preheat oven to 375°F (190°C, gas mark 5). Whisk the egg, sugar, and oil together in a bowl. Mix the lemon peel and all of the dry ingredientstogether in a separate bowl and stir with a wooden spoon until all of them are evenly dispersed throughout. Slowly add the dry ingredients into the egg, sugar, and oil, and mix to create a thick dough. Add the milk and mix well. Coat a baking sheet with nonstick vegetable oil spray. Scoop up tablespoons of the dough and drop them one by one in mounds onto the baking sheet, leaving 2 inches (5 cm) of space between. Bake for 15 to 20 minutes, just until the crust is barely golden brown and the dough is dry. Remove from the oven and let cool for 10 minutes. With a fork, mix the

lemon topping ingredients until the sugar is completely melded in. Drizzle 1 tablespoon ever each scone.

Yield: 10 servings

Each with: 21 g water; 218 calories (36% from fat, 8% from protein, 56% from carb); 5 g protein; 9 g total fat; 1 g saturated fat; 5 g monounsaturated fat; 3 g polyunsaturated fat; 32 g carb; 3 g fiber; 14 g sugar; 165 mg phosphorus; 138 mg calcium; 1 mg iron; 164 mg sodium; 152 mg potassium; 61 IU vitamin A; 16 mg vitamin E; 2 mg vitamin C; 21 mg cholesterol

12 Granola

Some healthy cereals are available if you are careful about reading the ingredient labels. But it would be hard to find one healthier or tastier than this homemade granola.

6 cups (48O g) rolled oats6 cups rolled wheat

2 cups (29O g) sunflower seeds 4 ounces (11C g) sesame seeds 2 cups (19O g) peanuts cups (255 g) coconut 1 cup (112 g) wheat germ 1½ cups (C55 ml) canola oil1 cup (C4O g) honey

½ cup (17O g) molasses 1 tablespoon (15 ml) vanilla extract 1 cup (145 g) raisins

Mix all dry ingredients together in large bowl. Put aside. Heat the oil,honey, molasses, and vanilla together and mix with dry ingredients. Spread mixture on baking sheets. Bake at 350°F (180°C, gas mark 4) for 30 to 40 minutes or until light brown. Stir frequently to brown evenly. Remove from oven and add raisins or any other dried fruit.

Yield: 30 servings

Each with: 10 g water; 391 calories (49% from fat, 8% from protein, 43% from carb); 8 g protein; 22 g total fat; 4 g saturated fat; 9 g monounsaturated fat; 8 g polyunsaturated fat; 44 g carb; 5 g fiber; 18 g sugar; 290 mg phosphorus; 75 mg calcium; 5 mg iron; 75 mg sodium; 372 mg potassium; 205IU vitamin A; 60 mg vitamin E; 1 mg vitamin C; 0 mg cholesterol

13 Toasty Nut Granola

This is great both as a snack or breakfast cereal.

6 cups (480 g) rolled oats

1 cup (110 g) chopped pecans

¾ cup (84 g) wheat germ

½ cup (115 g) firmly packed brown sugar

½ cup (40 g) shredded coconut

½ cup (72 g) sesame seeds

½ cup (120 ml) canola oil

½ cup (170 g) honey

1½ teaspoons vanilla extract

Toast oats in a 9 × 13-inch (23 × 33 cm) pan at 350°F (180°C, gas mark 4) for 10 minutes. Combine remaining ingredients in a large bowl and add toasted oats. Bake on 2 baking sheets at 350°F (180°C, gas mark 4) for 20 to 25 minutes. Stir when cool and store in refrigerator.

Yield: 28 servings

Each with: 4 g water; 194 calories (44% from fat, 9% from protein, 47% from carb); 5 g protein; 10 g total fat; 2 g saturated fat; 4 g monounsaturated fat; 4 g polyunsaturated fat; 24 g carb; 3 g fiber; 9 g sugar; 146 mg phosphorus; 42 mg calcium; 2 mg iron; 3 mg sodium; 139 mg potassium; 6 IU vitamin A; 0 mg vitamin E; 0 mg vitamin C; 0 mg cholesterol

14 Breakfast Bars

These contain a little more nutrition than commercial granola bars and are equally good for a breakfast on the run.

1 cup (8O g) quick-cooking oats

½ cup (6O g) whole wheat flour

½ cup (58 g) crunchy wheat-barley cereal, such as Grape-Nuts

½ teaspoon cinnamon1 egg

¼ cup (6O g) applesauce

¼ cup (85 g) honey

C tablespoons (45 g) brown sugar2 tablespoons (28 ml) canola oil

¼ cup (C6 g) sunflower seeds, unsalted

¼ cup (CO g) chopped walnuts 7 ounces (198 g) dried fruit

Preheat oven to 325°F (170°C, gas mark 3). Line a 9-inch (23 cm) square baking pan with aluminum foil. Spray the foil with nonstick vegetable oil spray. In a large bowl, stir together the oats, flour, cereal, and cinnamon. Add the egg, applesauce, honey, brown sugar, and oil. Mix well. Stir in the sunflower seeds, walnuts, and dried fruit. Spread mixture evenly in the prepared pan. Bake 30 minutes or until firm and lightly browned around the edges. Let cool. Use the foil to lift from the pan. Cut into bars and store in the refrigerator.

Yield: 12 servings

Each with: 16 g water; 222 calories (26% from fat, 9% from protein, 65% from carb); 6 g protein; 7 g total fat; 1 g saturated fat; 2 g monounsaturated fat; 3 g polyunsaturated fat; 38 g carb; 4 g fiber; 10 g sugar; 164 mg phosphorus; 27 mg calcium; 3 mg iron; 43 mg sodium; 284 mg potassium; 492 IU vitamin A; 6 mg vitamin E; 1 mg vitamin C; 20 mg cholesterol

15 Whole Wheat Coffee Cake

This is a nice whole wheat coffee cake with a crunchy filling.

1¾ cups (210 g) whole wheat pastry flour 1 teaspoon baking powder

1 teaspoon baking soda

½ cup (112 g) unsalted butter, softenedcup (1CC g) sugar

2 eggs

1 teaspoon vanilla extract1 cup (2CO g) sour cream Bran Nut Filling

⅓ cup (75 g) packed brown sugar

½ cup bran flakes (2O g) cereal

½ cup (6O g) chopped walnuts 1 teaspoon cinnamon

Mix flour, baking powder, and baking soda; set aside. In large bowl beat butter, sugar, eggs, and vanilla until light and fluffy. At low speed stir in sour cream alternately with flour mixture until blended. To make the bran nut filling, combine all filling ingredients in a small bowl. To assemble the cake, spread one-third of the sour cream mixture in a 9-inch (23 cm) square pan coated with nonstick vegetable oil spray. Sprinkle on about ½ cup filling. Repeat layering twice. Bake in preheated 350°F (180°C, gas mark 4) oven for 30 to 45 minutes. Cool slightly.

Yield: 12 servings

Each with: 27 g water; 275 calories (45% from fat, 8% from protein, 46% from carb); 6 g protein; 14 g total fat; 7 g saturated fat; 4 g monounsaturated fat; 2 g polyunsaturated fat; 33 g carb; 3 g fiber;

17 g sugar; 148 mg phosphorus; 68 mg calcium; 2 mg iron; 85 mg sodium; 174 mg potassium; 451 IU vitamin A; 97 mg vitamin E; 1 mg vitamin C; 68 mg cholesterol

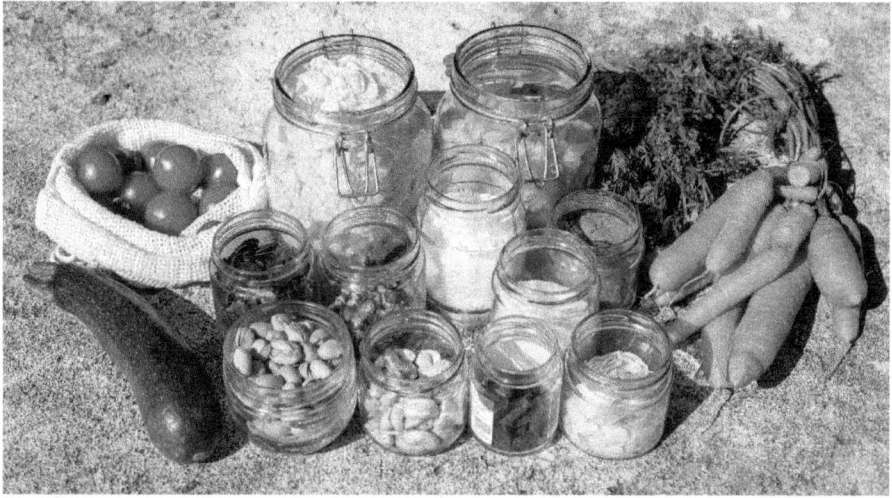

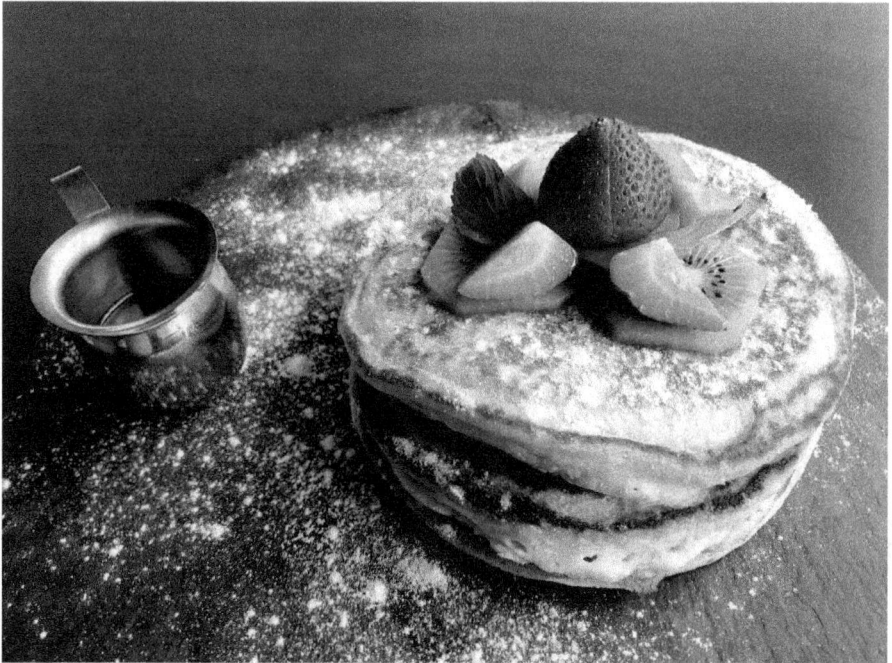

Main Dishes

Moving into main dishes, we start with legumes. You probably think of chili immediately. And we have some chili recipes, but we also have a variety of other soups, casseroles, and main-dish salads containing a wide variety of different kinds of beans.

16 Chicken Chili Verde

Here is yet another chili variation. Called "green chili" in Spanish, it does not contain tomatoes and has chicken instead of the more traditional beef. If you can't find cannellini beans, which are an Italian white kidney bean, youcan substitute any other white bean, such as navy or great northern beans.

C cups (COO g) cooked cannellini beans, drained 1 cup (16O g) chopped onion

½ teaspoon minced garlic

4 ounces (115 g) chopped chiles

2 teaspoons oregano1½ teaspoons cumin
¼ teaspoon ground cloves

¼ teaspoon cayenne

C cups (42O g) cooked diced chicken

2 cups (47O ml) low-sodium chicken broth

Combine all ingredients in a large pot and simmer gently about 1 hour.

Yield: 6 servings

Each with: 146 g water; 259 calories (20% from fat, 44% from protein, 36% from carb); 28 g protein; 6 g total fat; 2 g saturated fat; 2 g monounsaturated fat; 1 g polyunsaturated fat; 24 g carb; 7 g fiber; 2 g sugar; 303 mg phosphorus; 91 mg calcium; 4 mg iron; 66 mg sodium; 637 mg potassium; 322 IU vitamin A; 11 mg vitamin E; 49 mg vitamin C; 62 mg cholesterol

17 Pork Chop and Bean Skillet

This makes a good dinner with fried potatoes.

6 center-cut pork chops

1 tablespoon (15 ml) olive oil 1 cup (16O g) chopped onion

½ teaspoon minced garlic

½ cup (12O ml) low-sodium chicken broth

½ cup (125 g) barbecue sauce 2 jalapeño peppers, chopped

4 cups (684 g) no-salt-added pinto beans, drained

In a large skillet, sear pork chops in oil until brown, about 5 minutes. Remove pork chops and place on plate. Add onion and garlic to skillet; cook 10 minutes. Stir in broth, barbecue sauce, jalapeños, and beans. Heat mixture to a boil. Return pork to skillet. Reduce heat. Cover and simmer 50 to 60 minutes, stirring sauce and turning chops occasionally until meat is fork-tender.

Yield: 6 servings

Each with: 171 g water; 401 calories (23% from fat, 33% from protein, 43% from carb); 34 gprotein; 10 g total fat; 3 g saturated fat; 5 g monounsaturated fat; 1 g polyunsaturated fat; 43 g carb; 11 g fiber; 9 g sugar; 370 mg phosphorus; 76 mg calcium; 3 mg iron; 269 mg sodium; 874 mg potassium; 43 IU vitamin A; 1 mg vitamin E; 6 mg vitamin C; 63 mg cholesterol

18 Bean Balls

These are a vegetarian alternative to meatballs. If you are skeptical, youreally should try these.

1½ cups (265 g) cooked great northern beans, drained1 cup (115 g) whole wheat bread crumbs

1 tablespoon grated Parmesan cheese2 eggs

2 tablespoons parsley

2 teaspoons onion powder

Mash beans and add rest of ingredients. Form into balls and steam for 20 minutes. Serve with spaghetti as a substitute for meatballs.

Yield: 6 servings

Each with: 62 g water; 180 calories (17% from fat, 22% from protein, 61% from carb); 10 g protein;

3 g total fat; 1 g saturated fat; 1 g monounsaturated fat; 1 g polyunsaturated fat; 28 g carb; 4 g fiber; 2

g sugar; 165 mg phosphorus; 94 mg calcium; 2 mg iron; 71 mg sodium; 306 mg potassium; 201 IU vitamin A; 27 mg vitamin E; 3 mg vitamin C; 80 mg cholesterol

19 Chickpea Sandwich Spread

Are you looking for something a little different for a sandwich? Try this along with lettuce and tomato on a whole grain bread.

1½ cups (246 g) cooked chickpeas, drained (save juice)

½ teaspoon onion powder cup (CO g) chopped chives

1½ tablespoons (24 g) no-salt-added tomato paste teaspoon lemon juice

Mash chickpeas and mix with rest of ingredients. Add 1/3 cup of the reserved juice and process in a blender or food processor. Use as sandwich spread.

Yield: 6 servings

Each with: 50 g water; 77 calories (8% from fat, 17% from protein, 75% from carb); 3 g protein; 1 g total fat; 0 g saturated fat; 0 g monounsaturated fat; 0 g polyunsaturated fat; 15 g carb; 3 g fiber; 1 g sugar; 61 mg phosphorus; 26 mg calcium; 1 mg iron; 184 mg sodium; 162 mg potassium; 309 IU vitamin A; 0 mg vitamin E; 6 mg vitamin C; 0 mg cholesterol

20 Italian Baked Beans

Here is an Italian-flavored version of baked beans.

1 pound (455 g) navy beans

8 cups (1.9 L) water

1 pound (455 g) hot Italian sausage links, sliced 1 cup (16O g) chopped onion

   ¹/₃ıp (5O g) green bell pepper, cut in 1-inch (2.5 cm) pieces

½ cup (C5 g) halved mushrooms2 bay leaves

   ¹/₃ıp (8O ml) ketchupcup (11C g) molasses

1 t¹/₃blespoon dry mustard

2 teaspoons crushed oregano

½ teaspoon black pepper

¼ teaspoon garlic salt

Rinse beans; place in large saucepan. Add water. Bring to boil; reduce heat and simmer, covered, for 1 hour. Transfer to bowl; cover and refrigerate overnight. Drain beans, reserving 1½ cups of the liquid. In slow cooker, combine drained beans, sausage, onion, bell pepper, mushrooms, and bay leaves. Blend reserved bean liquid with ketchup, molasses, mustard, oregano, pepper, and garlic salt; stir into bean mixture. Cover and cook on high heat for 6 hours or on low heat for 12 hours.

Yield: 8 servings

Each with: 310 g water; 452 calories (37% from fat, 17% from protein, 45% from carb); 20 g protein; 19 g total fat; 7 g saturated fat; 8 g monounsaturated fat; 3 g polyunsaturated fat; 52 g carb; 9 g fiber; 13 g sugar; 331 mg phosphorus; 142 mg calcium; 5 mg iron; 433 mg sodium; 1125 mg potassium; 141 IU vitamin A; 0 mg vitamin E; 11 mg vitamin C; 43 mg cholesterol

21 White Bean and Tuna Salad

This makes a great luncheon salad. It can also be a main dish in somewhatlarger portions.

2 cups (2OO g) cooked cannellini beans, drained and rinsed1C ounces (C68 g) tuna, drained

1 cup (18O g) seeded, diced tomato

½ cup (8O g) chopped red onion

2 tablespoons (CO ml) lemon juice C teaspoons (15 ml) Dijon mustard

⅓p (8O ml) olive oil

¼ cup chopped fresh basil

Combine beans, tuna, tomato, and onion in large bowl. Combine lemon juice and mustard in small bowl. Gradually whisk in olive oil. Add to salad.Mix in basil.

Yield: 4 servings

Each with: 192 g water; 406 calories (47% from fat, 29% from protein, 24% from carb); 30 gprotein; 21 g total fat; 3 g saturated fat; 14 g monounsaturated fat; 3 g polyunsaturated fat; 24 g carb; 8 g fiber; 2 g sugar; 375 mg phosphorus; 129 mg calcium; 4 mg iron; 303 mg sodium; 769 mg potassium; 530 IU vitamin A; 6 mg vitamin E; 12 mg vitamin C; 39 mg cholesterol

22 Beef and Barley Stew

This hearty stew is a full meal in a bowl (although I prefer it with a slice offresh hot bread).

1½ pounds (675 g) beef round steak

¼ cup (C1 g) flour

2 tablespoons (28 ml) olive oil 1 cup (16O g) chopped onion

½ teaspoon crushed garlic

C cups (71O ml) low-sodium beef broth2 cups (26O g) sliced carrot

¼ cup (5O g) pearl barley

1 tablespoon (15 ml) soy sauce

½ teaspoon oregano

½ cup (5O g) chopped celery

½ teaspoon black pepper

Trim fat from meat and cut into bite-size cubes. Dust beef with flour. Usinga heavy pot, brown beef in hot oil, browning all sides. Remove meat and set aside. Add onion and garlic to drippings and cook until onion is transparent. Return the meat to pot. Add broth, barley, soy sauce, and oregano. Cover and simmer for 45 minutes. Add carrot and simmer until meat is tender, about 40 minutes. Add water as needed. Season with pepper.

Yield: 6 servings

Each with: 257 g water; 352 calories (28% from fat, 52% from protein, 20% from carb); 45 g protein; 11 g total fat; 3 g saturated fat; 6 g monounsaturated fat; 1 g polyunsaturated fat; 17 g carb; 3 g fiber; 3 g sugar; 327 mg phosphorus; 42 mg calcium; 5 mg iron; 310 mg sodium; 693 mg potassium; 7222 IU vitamin A; 0 mg vitamin E; 5 mg vitamin C; 102 mg cholesterol

23 Beef Barley Skillet

This tasty and healthy family meal cooks in only one pan.

¾ pound (CC8 g) ground beef

½ cup (8O g) chopped onion

¼ cup (C8 g) chopped green bell pepper

¼ cup (25 g) chopped celery

¼ teaspoon black pepper

½ teaspoon marjoram1 teaspoon sugar
1 teaspoon Worcestershire sauce

2 cups (48O g) no-salt-added canned tomatoes, broken up1½ cups (C55 ml) water
¾ cup (15O g) pearl barley

Sauté meat, onion, green pepper, and celery in nonstick fry pan. Drain off excess fat; stir in remaining ingredients. Bring to a boil. Reduce heat to simmer; cover and cook about 1 hour.

Yield: 3 servings

Each with: 389 g water; 477 calories (21% from fat, 31% from protein, 48% from carb); 29 g protein; 9 g total fat; 3 g saturated fat; 3 g monounsaturated fat; 1 g polyunsaturated fat; 45 g carb; 10g fiber; 7 g sugar; 326 mg phosphorus; 90 mg calcium; 6 mg iron; 129 mg sodium; 932 mg potassium; 292 IU vitamin A; 0 mg vitamin E; 30 mg vitamin C; 78 mg cholesterol

24 Stroganoff

Up the fiber in your stroganoff by using whole wheat noodles.

½ pound (225 g) ground beef, extra lean

½ cup (C5 g) sliced mushrooms1 packet onion soup mix

1 tablespoon whole wheat flour1¾ cups (414 ml) water

8 ounces (225 g) whole wheat noodles, cooked and drained8 tablespoons (12O g) plain fat-free yogurt
Brown beef and drain. Add mushrooms. Whisk dry soup mix and flour into water and heat. Stir until thickened. Combine thickened onion soup and cooked beef. Serve over whole wheat noodles. Garnish with a dollop of yogurt.

Yield: 4 servings

Each with: 178 g water; 360 calories (26% from fat, 23% from protein, 51% from carb); 21 g protein; 11 g total fat; 4 g saturated fat; 4 g monounsaturated fat; 1 g polyunsaturated fat; 48 g carb; 2 g fiber; 3 g sugar; 288 mg phosphorus; 95 mg calcium; 3 mg iron; 222 mg sodium; 397 mg potassium; 2 IU vitamin A; 1 mg vitamin E; 1 mg vitamin C; 40 mg cholesterol

25 Western Casserole

This simple beef-and-noodle casserole is updated to give you more fiberwithout sacrificing taste.

1 pound (455 g) beef stew meat, cut in cubes

¼ cup (CO g) whole wheat flour

¼ cup (6O ml) olive oil

6 ounces (17O g) no-salt-added tomato paste

½ cup (12O ml) dry red wine1 cup (2C5 ml) water
1 teaspoon thyme

1 teaspoon oregano

1 cup (7O g) sliced mushrooms 1 cup (18O g) chopped tomato
4 ounces (115 g) whole wheat noodles, cooked and drained1 cup (115 g) shredded Cheddar cheese

Coat meat with flour; brown in oil. Add all ingredients except noodles and cheese. Cover and simmer for 1 hour. Add noodles and cheese. Simmer 5 minutes more and serve.

Yield: 4 servings

Each with: 264 g water; 607 calories (47% from fat, 27% from protein, 26% from carb); 41 gprotein; 31 g total fat; 11 g saturated fat; 15 g monounsaturated fat; 2 g polyunsaturated fat; 39 gcarb; 3 g fiber; 6 g sugar; 563 mg phosphorus; 299 mg calcium; 6 mg iron; 341 mg sodium; 1114 mg potassium; 1239 IU vitamin A; 85 mg vitamin E; 20 mg vitamin C; 96 mg cholesterol

26 Chicken Barley Chowder

This simple, creamy soup of chicken and barley is perfect for a cold day.

2 tablespoons (28 ml) olive oil

½ cup (6O g) minced celery

**¾ cup (12O g) minced onion1 tablespoon flour
½ teaspoon black pepper**

6 cups (1.4 L) low-sodium chicken broth 1 cup (2OO g) pearl barley

1 pound (455 g) cooked boneless chicken breast, shredded

½ cup (12O ml) fat-free evaporated milk

Heat oil in heavy saucepan. Sauté celery and onion; sprinkle with flour and pepper. Gradually stir in broth and barley. Add chicken. Simmer covered for about an hour, stirring occasionally until barley is tender. Remove from heat and add milk.

Yield: 4 servings

Each with: 499 g water; 452 calories (23% from fat, 37% from protein, 41% from carb); 42 g protein; 12 g total fat; 2 g saturated fat; 6 g monounsaturated fat; 2 g polyunsaturated fat; 47 g carb; 9 g fiber; 6 g sugar; 528 mg phosphorus; 148 mg calcium; 4 mg iron; 236 mg sodium; 995 mg potassium; 218 IU vitamin A; 45 mg vitamin E; 4 mg vitamin C; 67 mg cholesterol

27 Chicken Barley Soup

This is a nice change from chicken and noodle or chicken and rice soup thatfeatures barley.

C pound (1¼ kg) chicken, cut up 2 quarts (1.9 L) water

1½ cups (195 g) diced carrot 1 cup (12O g) diced celery

1 cup (2OO g) pearl barley

½ cup (6O g) chopped onion 1 bay leaf

½ teaspoon poultry seasoning

½ teaspoon black pepper

½ teaspoon dried sage

Cook chicken in water until tender. Cool broth and skim off fat. Bone chicken and cut into bite-size pieces; return to kettle along with remaining ingredients. Return to heat and bring to a boil. Simmer covered for at least 1 hour until vegetables are tender and barley is done, adding more water if needed. Remove bay leaf and serve. **Yield:** 6 servings

Each with: 546 g water; 400 calories (18% from fat, 54% from protein, 28% from carb); 53 g protein; 8 g total fat; 2 g saturated fat; 2 g monounsaturated fat; 2 g polyunsaturated fat; 27 g carb; 7g fiber; 3 g sugar; 493 mg phosphorus; 69 mg calcium; 3 mg iron; 224 mg sodium; 829 mg potassium; 5595 IU vitamin A; 36 mg vitamin E; 9 mg vitamin C; 159 mg cholesterol

28 Chicken Chili with Barley

This is not your traditional chili. In fact, some might argue that it's not chili at all. But the flavor is great and it will be appreciated by anyone who likes Mexican or Tex-Mex cooking.

1 cup (16O g) chopped onion

½ teaspoon minced garlic

1 tablespoon (15 ml) olive oil

2 cups (475 ml) water

¾ cup (15O g) pearl barley

4 cups (1 kg) no-salt-added canned tomatoes2 cups (475 ml) low-sodium chicken broth
6 ounces (17O g) frozen corn

1 can jalapeño peppers, chopped1 tablespoon chili powder
½ teaspoon cumin

C cups (42O g) cubed cooked chicken

In a Dutch oven, cook onion and garlic in the oil until onion is tender. Add remaining ingredients except chicken. Bring to a boil. Reduce heat, cover, and simmer 10 minutes, stirring occasionally. Add chicken and continue simmering an additional 5 to 10 minutes until chicken is heated through and barley is tender.

Yield: 9 servings

Each with: 267 g water; 210 calories (26% from fat, 34% from protein, 41% from carb); 18 g protein; 6 g total fat; 1 g saturated fat; 2 g monounsaturated fat; 2 g polyunsaturated fat; 22 g carb; 5 g fiber; 4 g sugar; 194 mg phosphorus; 57 mg calcium; 3 mg iron; 86 mg sodium; 529 mg potassium; 453 IU vitamin A; 7 mg vitamin E; 14 mg vitamin C; 42 mg cholesterol

Side Dishes and Salads

Grains are a natural for side dishes. Rice is probably the one you think of first, but don't ignore other choices such as barley and bulgur. We've included a number of recipes here to get you thinking about them.

29 Mexican Rice

This family favorite is a quick and flavorful use for leftover rice.

1 cup (22O g) cooked brown rice 2 tablespoons (28 ml) olive oil

½ cup (8O g) chopped onion

¼ pound (11C g) shredded Cheddar cheese 1 jalapeño pepper, chopped

Brown rice in oil. Add remaining ingredients. Cover and simmer untilheated through and cheese is melted.

Yield: 4 servings

Each with: 67 g water; 237 calories (63% from fat, 14% from protein, 23% from carb); 9 g protein; 17 g total fat; 7 g saturated fat; 8 g monounsaturated fat; 1 g polyunsaturated fat; 14 g carb; 1 g fiber; 1 g sugar; 192 mg phosphorus; 214 mg calcium; 1 mg iron; 179 mg sodium; 86 mg potassium; 312 IU vitamin A; 73 mg vitamin E; 3 mg vitamin C; 30 mg cholesterol

30 Tomato Pilaf

This makes a delicious side dish for any meal where you would normallyhave rice or noodles.

2 cups (48O g) no-salt-added canned tomatoes 2 teaspoons (1O ml) olive oil

½ cup (8O g) minced onion1 cup (14O g) bulgur

½ cup (CO g) chopped fresh parsley

Drain tomatoes, reserving juice. Heat oil in a skillet and add onion. Sauté until tender. Add bulgur and brown for 1 minute until golden colored. Put in casserole dish. Add enough water to reserved tomato juice to make 2 cups (475 ml) liquid. Pour over wheat mixture along with parsley and tomatoes. Cover. Bake at 350°F (180°C, gas mark 4) for 45 minutes. Remove cover; stir and bake, uncovered, 5 minutes longer.

Yield: 4 servings

Each with: 141 g water; 171 calories (14% from fat, 12% from protein, 73% from carb); 6 g protein;

3 g total fat; 0 g saturated fat; 2 g monounsaturated fat; 1 g polyunsaturated fat; 34 g carb; 8 g fiber; 4

g sugar; 138 mg phosphorus; 64 mg calcium; 3 mg iron; 27 mg sodium; 440 mg potassium; 776 IU vitamin A; 0 mg vitamin E; 23 mg vitamin C; 0 mg cholesterol

31 Rice and Cheese Casserole

This cheesy rice side dish is a good use for leftover rice. And it is good enough that you may want to make sure some of it is left over.

2 cups (44O g) cooked brown rice

1 cup (115 g) shredded Cheddar cheese 2 tablespoons (2O g) chopped onion

C eggs, slightly beaten

Place rice in a 1½-quart (1.5 L) baking dish. Combine remaining ingredients and pour over rice. Bake at 350°F (180°C, gas mark 4) for 25 minutes.

Yield: 4 servings

Each with: 120 g water; 303 calories (48% from fat, 21% from protein, 31% from carb); 16 g protein; 16 g total fat; 8 g saturated fat; 5 g monounsaturated fat; 1 g polyunsaturated fat; 24 g carb; 2 g fiber; 1 g sugar; 332 mg phosphorus; 271 mg calcium; 1 mg iron; 269 mg sodium; 138 mg potassium; 535 IU vitamin A; 144 mg vitamin E; 0 mg vitamin C; 212 mg cholesterol

32 Southern Rice Pilaf

This rice has lots of good things added to it.

2 cups (C8O g) brown rice

4 tablespoons (55 g) unsalted butter, melted

½ teaspoon cumin seeds

¼ teaspoon cinnamon2 whole cloves
1 cup (15O g) peas

C½ cups (8CO ml) water

½ cup (8O g) finely sliced onion

¼ cup (27 g) slivered almonds

¼ cup (C5 g) raisins

Wash rice, drain, and set aside for about 30 minutes. Put half the butter in a saucepan, add the cumin seeds, and heat. When cumin seeds turn slightly brown, add cinnamon and cloves and the peas. Fry for a minute and add the rice. Mix for another minute. Add the water and after it starts to boil, cover and put on low heat and cook until done, about 35 to 45 minutes. For garnish, take half the remaining butter and fry the onion until lightly brown and sprinkle on top of rice. With the rest of the butter, fry slivered almonds and raisins until lightly brown and sprinkle on top of the onion and rice. Serve hot.

Yield: 4 servings

Each with: 332 g water; 333 calories (45% from fat, 8% from protein, 47% from carb); 7 g protein; 17 g total fat; 8 g saturated fat; 6 g monounsaturated fat; 2 g polyunsaturated fat; 40 g carb; 6 g fiber; 10 g sugar; 180 mg phosphorus; 66 mg calcium; 2 mg iron; 144 mg sodium; 291 mg potassium; 1199 IU vitamin A; 95 mg vitamin E; 6 mg vitamin C; 31 mg cholesterol

33 Barley and Pine Nut Casserole

This is a simple but flavorful side dish with the additional crunch of pine nuts. It's good with any grilled meat, especially ones with Italian seasoning.

1 cup (2OO g) pearl barley

½ cup (7O g) pine nuts, divided C tablespoons (42 g) unsalted butter, divided 1 cup (16O g) chopped onion ½ cup (CO g) minced fresh parsley

¼ cup (25 g) minced scallions ¼ teaspoon black pepper, freshly ground C cups (C55 ml) low-sodium chicken broth, heated to boiling

Preheat oven to 375°F (190°C, gas mark 5). Rinse and drain barley. Toast pine nuts in 1 tablespoon butter in a skillet. Remove nuts with slotted spoon and set aside. Add remaining butter to skillet with onion and barley and stir until toasted. Stir in nuts, parsley, scallions, and pepper. Spoon into a 1½- quart (1.5 L) casserole dish. Pour hot broth over casserole and mix well. Bake uncovered for 1 hour and 15 minutes.

Yield: 6 servings

Each with: 152 g water; 268 calories (48% from fat, 12% from protein, 41% from carb); 8 g protein; 15 g total fat; 5 g saturated fat; 4 g monounsaturated fat; 5 g polyunsaturated fat; 29 g carb; 6 g fiber; 2 g sugar; 196 mg phosphorus; 35 mg calcium; 2 mg iron; 45 mg sodium; 390 mg potassium; 651 IU vitamin A; 48 mg vitamin E; 10 mg vitamin C; 15 mg cholesterol

34 Barley Casserole

This barley casserole is flavored with beef broth, making it a great choice to have with steak or roast beef.

½ cup (8O g) chopped onion

2 tablespoons (28 ml) olive oil2 cups (4OO g) pearl barley

6 cups (1.4 L) low-sodium beef broth

¼ teaspoon black pepper

1 cup (2C5 ml) boiling water

Sauté onion in oil until transparent. Add barley and continue cooking until barley is lightly browned. Put in 2-quart (2 L) casserole dish that has been sprayed with nonstick vegetable oil spray. Just before baking, bring broth to a boil. Add broth, pepper, and water to barley and stir gently. Bake covered 1 hour or until barley is tender. Add more water or broth if necessary.

Yield: 8 servings

Each with: 218 g water; 209 calories (20% from fat, 15% from protein, 65% from carb); 8 g protein;
5 g total fat; 1 g saturated fat; 3 g monounsaturated fat; 1 g polyunsaturated fat; 35 g carb; 8 g fiber; 1
g sugar; 148 mg phosphorus; 29 mg calcium; 2 mg iron; 112 mg sodium; 320 mg potassium; 13 IU vitamin A; 0 mg vitamin E; 1 mg vitamin C; 0 mg cholesterol

35 Barley Mushroom Pilaf

This is a quick and easy way to give barley some extra flavor. We like this with chicken, but it would go with a number of meals.

2 teaspoons (1O ml) olive oil

½ cup (C5 g) sliced mushrooms 1 cup (2OO g) pearl barley

C cups (71O ml) low-sodium chicken broth 2 tablespoons chopped scallions

¼ teaspoon rosemary

2 tablespoons grated Parmesan cheese

Heat olive oil in saucepan; add mushrooms and sauté until limp. Add barley, broth, scallions, and rosemary. Bring to a boil. Reduce heat to low, cover, and cook 45 minutes or until barley is tender and liquid is absorbed. Sprinkle Parmesan cheese over pilaf and serve.

Yield: 4 servings

Each with: 189 g water; 228 calories (20% from fat, 18% from protein, 62% from carb); 11 g protein; 5 g total fat; 1 g saturated fat; 3 g monounsaturated fat; 1 g polyunsaturated fat; 37 g carb; 8 g fiber; 1 g sugar; 207 mg phosphorus; 60 mg calcium; 2 mg iron; 108 mg sodium; 403 mg potassium; 56 IU vitamin A; 4 mg vitamin E; 1 mg vitamin C; 3 mg cholesterol

36 Barley Risotto

This is not exactly like traditional risotto, but it's still a delightful side dish.

½ cup (1OO g) pearl barley 1 teaspoon (5 ml) olive oil

C tablespoons (21 g) minced carrot C tablespoons (CO g) minced onion C tablespoons (24 g) minced celery1 teaspoon rosemary 1 bay leaf

½ teaspoon black pepper

1½ cups (C55 ml) vegetable broth

Put barley in heavy skillet over low heat and toast. Shake pan frequently. When barley turns light brown and smells nutty, about 15 to 20 minutes, remove from skillet. Heat oil in skillet, add minced vegetables, and sauté for 3 minutes. Add barley and stir to coat grains. Add herbs and broth. Simmer, covered, until barley is tender and liquid is absorbed, about 35 minutes. Remove bay leaf before serving.

Yield: 4 servings

Each with: 108 g water; 138 calories (24% from fat, 11% from protein, 65% from carb); 4 g protein;
4 g total fat; 1 g saturated fat; 2 g monounsaturated fat; 1 g polyunsaturated fat; 23 g carb; 5 g fiber; 1
g sugar; 87 mg phosphorus; 27 mg calcium; 1 mg iron; 450 mg sodium; 187 mg potassium; 1041 IU vitamin A; 0 mg vitamin E; 3 mg vitamin C; 0 mg cholesterol

37 Bulgur Pilaf

This simple dish can be used as a side dish similar to cooked rice.

2 tablespoons (28 ml) olive oil

½ cup (5O g) chopped celery 1 cup (16O g) chopped onion

1 cup (7O g) sliced mushrooms 1 cup (14O g) bulgur

½ teaspoon dried dill

¼ teaspoon dried oregano

¼ teaspoon black pepper, fresh ground

2 cups (475 ml) low-sodium chicken broth

Heat oil in a large skillet; add celery, onion, and mushrooms. Stir constantly until vegetables are tender. Add bulgur and cook until golden. Add seasonings and chicken broth. Cover and bring to a boil. Reduce heat and simmer 15 minutes.

Yield: 6 servings

Each with: 122 g water; 148 calories (31% from fat, 13% from protein, 56% from carb); 5 g protein;
5 g total fat; 1 g saturated fat; 4 g monounsaturated fat; 1 g polyunsaturated fat; 22 g carb; 5 g fiber; 2
g sugar; 114 mg phosphorus; 24 mg calcium; 1 mg iron; 37 mg sodium; 267 mg potassium; 49 IU vitamin A; 0 mg vitamin E; 3 mg vitamin C; 0 mg cholesterol

38 Bulgur Wheat with Squash

Sometimes grain side dishes can be pretty plain. This one gets it flavor from butternut squash, and it turns out to be a winning combination.

1½ tablespoons (21 g) unsalted butter

½ cup (8O g) chopped onion

1 cup (14O g) peeled and cubed butternut squash

½ cup (7O g) bulgur2 whole cloves
2 cinnamon sticks

1 bay leaf

1 cup (2C5 ml) low-sodium chicken broth

Melt butter over medium heat. Add onion and squash. Cook until onion is soft. Add bulgur, cloves, cinnamon, and bay leaf. Stir until bulgur is brown. Stir in chicken broth. Cover and bring to a boil. Reduce heat and cook 15 minutes. Remove spices before serving.

Yield: 4 servings

Each with: 108 g water; 131 calories (32% from fat, 11% from protein, 57% from carb); 4 g protein;
5 g total fat; 3 g saturated fat; 1 g monounsaturated fat; 0 g polyunsaturated fat; 20 g carb; 4 g fiber; 2
g sugar; 89 mg phosphorus; 31 mg calcium; 1 mg iron; 24 mg sodium; 277 mg potassium; 3855 IUvitamin A; 36 mg vitamin E; 9 mg vitamin C; 11 mg cholesterol

39 Stuffed Tomatoes

Tomatoes stuffed with a rice/cheese/veggie mix make a nice side dish for just about any kind of meat.

6 medium tomatoes

2 tablespoons (28 ml) olive oil cup (CC g) chopped celery

2 tablespoons (2O g) chopped onion 2 cups (44O g) cooked brown rice

¼ cup (25 g) grated Parmesan cheese 1 tablespoon chopped fresh parsley

1 teaspoon basil teaspoon black pepper te⅛spoon garlic powder

Cut a thin slice from the top of each tomato. Set tops aside. Scoop out center of tomatoes; chop pulp, and set aside. Place shells upside down on paper towels to drain. Lightly oil 9-inch (23 cm) pie plate or round baking dish. Place tomatoes in dish. Cover with aluminum foil. Preheat oven to 350°F (180°C, gas mark 4). Heat oil in medium saucepan. Add celery and onion. Sauté over moderate heat until celery is tender. Remove from heat. Add reserved tomato pulp, rice, cheese, parsley, basil, pepper, and garlic powder; mix well. Fill tomato shells with rice mixture. Replace tomato tops, if desired. Bake at 350°F (180°C, gas mark 4), 30 to 45 minutes or until tomatoes are tender.

Yield: 6 servings

Each with: 197 g water; 164 calories (36% from fat, 11% from protein, 53% from carb); 5 g protein;

7 g total fat; 2 g saturated fat; 4 g monounsaturated fat; 1 g polyunsaturated fat; 23 g carb; 3 g fiber; 1

g sugar; 124 mg phosphorus; 67 mg calcium; 1 mg iron; 86 mg sodium; 392 mg potassium; 1036 IUvitamin A; 5 mg vitamin E; 40 mg vitamin C; 4 mg cholesterol

40 Rigatoni with Artichoke Sauce

This is a nice pasta sauce flavored with marinated artichoke hearts.

1 pound (455 g) whole wheat rigatoni

6 ounces (17O g) artichoke hearts, drained

¼ cup (6O ml) olive oil

¾ teaspoon minced garlic

2 tablespoons chopped fresh parsley

C cups (72O g) no-salt-added canned tomatoes, drained and choppedteaspoon red pepper flakes

¼ cup (25 g) grated Parmesan cheese

¼ teaspoon black pepper, fresh ground

Cook pasta according to directions. Meanwhile, slice artichokes thinly. In large saucepan, heat oil and sauté garlic 2 minutes. Add artichoke hearts, parsley, tomatoes, and pepper flakes. Cook 20 minutes, stirring occasionally. Drain rigatoni and place in serving dish. Top pasta with sauce and sprinkle with Parmesan cheese and black pepper.

Yield: 6 servings

Each with: 145 g water; 395 calories (25% from fat, 14% from protein, 61% from carb); 15 g protein; 12 g total fat; 2 g saturated fat; 7 g monounsaturated fat; 2 g polyunsaturated fat; 65 g carb; 3 g fiber; 3 g sugar; 267 mg phosphorus; 123 mg calcium; 4 mg iron; 101 mg sodium; 478 mg potassium; 326 IU vitamin A; 5 mg vitamin E; 14 mg vitamin C; 4 mg cholesterol

Breads

Whole grain breads and rolls are a great way to add extra fiber to your diet. We have a number of yeast bread recipes here that will help you do just that. But don't stop there; we also have recipes for whole grain biscuits and cornbread and for making your own higher-fiber tortillas, flatbread, pizza crust, and bagels.

41 Maple Oatmeal Bread

Being a slightly sweet bread with maple flavor, this one is just made for breakfast. It seems to me it would be perfect for French toast.

1¾ teaspoons yeast

cup (157 ml) warm water 2½ cups (C42 g) bread flour

½ cup (6O g) whole wheat flour cup (27 g) rolled oats

cu⅓(8O ml) maple syrup

¼ cup (17 g) nonfat dry milk

2 tablespoons (28 g) unsalted butter, room temperature

Add ingredients to the bread machine in the order

Yield: 12 servings

Each with: 21 g water; 178 calories (14% from fat, 12% from protein, 74% from carb); 6 g protein;

3 g total fat; 1 g saturated fat; 1 g monounsaturated fat; 0 g polyunsaturated fat; 33 g carb; 2 g fiber; 6

g sugar; 89 mg phosphorus; 32 mg calcium; 2 mg iron; 11 mg sodium; 129 mg potassium; 94 IU vitamin A; 26 mg vitamin E; 0 mg vitamin C; 5 mg cholesterol

42 German Dark Bread

To me this is almost purely a sandwich bread. Other than maybe a pork- chops-and-cabbage meal, I can't picture it for anything else. But it's perfect with mild-flavored fillings like chicken, turkey, or egg salad.

1 cup (2C5 ml) water

¼ cup (85 g) molasses

1 tablespoon unsalted butter 2 cups (274 g) bread flour 1¼ cups (16O g) rye flour
2 tablespoons cocoa powder 1½ teaspoons yeast
1 tablespoon vital wheat gluten

Place ingredients in bread machine in order specified by the manufacturer. Process on whole wheat cycle.

Yield: 12 servings

Each with: 25 g water; 156 calories (9% from fat, 11% from protein, 79% from carb); 5 g protein; 2 g total fat; 1 g saturated fat; 0 g monounsaturated fat; 0 g polyunsaturated fat; 31 g carb; 3 g fiber; 4 g sugar; 58 mg phosphorus; 22 mg calcium; 2 mg iron; 4 mg sodium; 175 mg potassium; 30 IU vitamin A; 8 mg vitamin E; 0 mg vitamin C; 3 mg cholesterol

43 Onion and Garlic Wheat Bread

Looking for a bread with a little more flavor to stand up to some of yourspicier meals? This may be just the one.

½ cup (8O g) finely chopped onion

½ teaspoon finely chopped garlic 1 tablespoon sugar

½ cup (6O g) whole wheat flour 2½ cups (C42 g) bread flour

1½ tablespoons nonfat dry milk1½ teaspoons yeast

¾ cup (175 ml) water

1½ tablespoons (21 g) unsalted butter

Place ingredients in bread machine in order specified by manufacturer. Process on white bread cycle.

Yield: 12 servings

Each with: 25 g water; 143 calories (13% from fat, 13% from protein, 74% from carb); 5 g protein;

2 g total fat; 1 g saturated fat; 0 g monounsaturated fat; 0 g polyunsaturated fat; 27 g carb; 2 g fiber; 2

g sugar; 59 mg phosphorus; 15 mg calcium; 2 mg iron; 5 mg sodium; 79 mg potassium; 58 IU vitamin A; 16 mg vitamin E; 1 mg vitamin C; 4 mg cholesterol

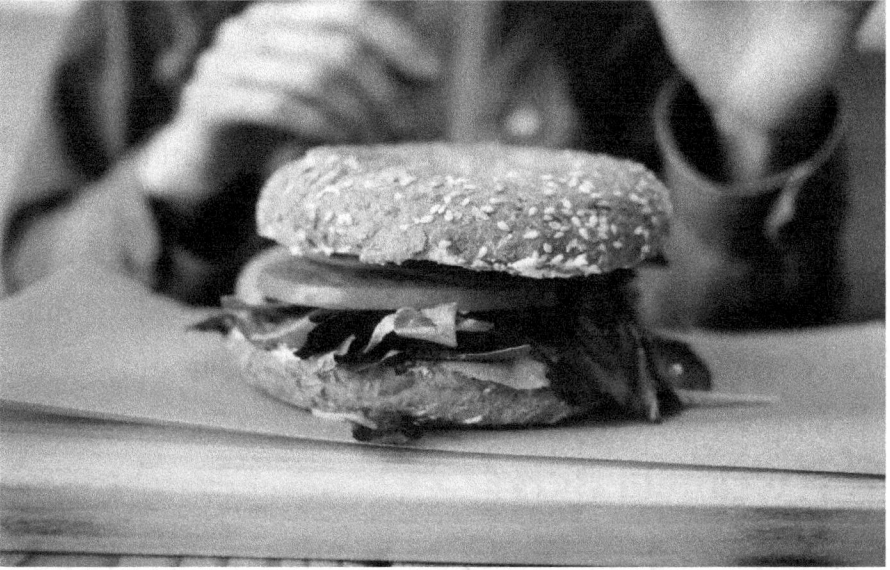

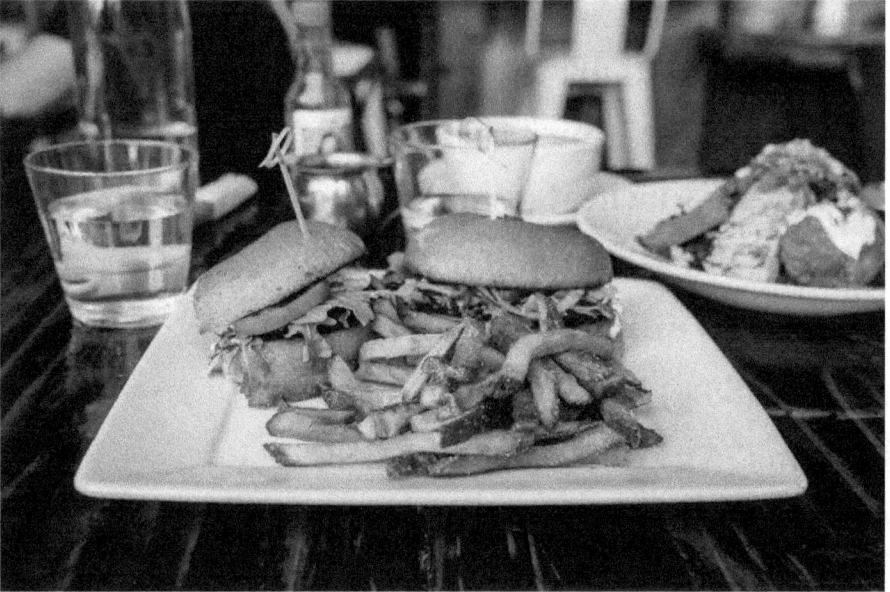

Desserts and Other Sweets

Yes, there actually are recipes for desserts made with legumes. Admittedly there aren't a lot, and a lot of them tend to be kind of similar, but I was so impressed with the whole idea that I decided to go ahead and make it a separate chapter, even if it does only contain two recipes. You really should try the bean pie—it will not be what you expect.

44 Granola Bars

You can add unsalted nuts to this if you want or substitute chocolate chips or other dried fruit for the raisins to vary the flavor.

C cups (240 g) quick-cooking oats

½ cup (115 g) brown sugar

¼ cup (28 g) wheat germ

½ cup (112 g) unsalted butter

¼ cup (60 ml) corn syrup

¼ cup (85 g) honey

½ cup (75 g) raisins

½ cup (40 g) sweetened coconut

Combine the oats, sugar, and wheat germ. Cut in the butter until the mixture is crumbly. Stir in the corn syrup and honey. Add the raisins and coconut. Press into a 9-inch (23 cm) square pan coated with nonstick vegetable oil spray. Bake in a 350°F (180°C, gas mark 4) oven for 20 to 25 minutes. Let cool 10 minutes and then cut into bars.

Yield: 27 servings

Each with: 4 g water; 153 calories (30% from fat, 8% from protein, 61% from carb); 3 g protein; 5 g total fat; 3 g saturated fat; 1 g monounsaturated fat; 1 g polyunsaturated fat; 24 g carb; 2 g fiber; 10 g sugar; 107 mg phosphorus; 17 mg calcium; 1 mg iron; 9 mg sodium; 129 mg potassium; 105 IUvitamin A; 28 mg vitamin E; 0 mg vitamin C; 9 mg cholesterol

45 Honey Oatmeal Cake

This makes a great breakfast or snack cake. Of course, I happen to be very fond of the flavor of honey.

1¼ cups (295 ml) water, boiling 1 cup (80 g) rolled oats

½ cup (112 g) unsalted butter, softened 1½ cups (510 g) honey

1 eggs

1 teaspoon vanilla extract

1¾ cups (210 g) whole wheat pastry flour 1 teaspoon baking soda

1 teaspoon ground cinnamon

¼ teaspoon ground nutmeg

Combine first 3 ingredients in a large bowl; stir well. Set aside for 20 minutes. Add honey, eggs, and vanilla; stir well. Combine whole wheat flour and remaining ingredients; gradually add to honey mixture. Pour into a greased and floured 13 × 9 × 2-inch (33 × 23 × 5 cm) baking pan. Bake at 350°F (180°C, gas mark 4) for 30 to 40 minutes or until toothpick comes out clean. Cool in pan. Frost if desired or sprinkle with confectioners' sugar.

Yield: 15 servings

Each with: 35 g water; 238 calories (27% from fat, 6% from protein,

67% from carb); 4 g protein; 8 g total fat; 4 g saturated fat; 2 g monounsaturated fat; 1 g polyunsaturated fat; 42 g carb; 2 g fiber; 28g sugar; 92 mg phosphorus; 18 mg calcium; 1 mg iron; 14 mg sodium; 107 mg potassium; 227 IU vitamin A; 61 mg vitamin E; 0 mg vitamin C; 48 mg cholesterol

46 Red Velvet Cake

This is one of those old-time traditional cakes, updated to provide a littleextra fiber by using whole wheat flour.

2½ cups (COO g) whole wheat pastry flour 1½ cups (COO g) sugar

2 teaspoons cocoa powder 1 teaspoon baking soda

2 eggs

½ cup (12O ml) canola oil

½ cup (12O ml) buttermilk

2 tablespoons (28 ml) red food coloring 1 teaspoon vanilla extract

Icing

¼ cup (55 g) unsalted butter

4 cups (4OO g) confectioners' sugar

½ teaspoon vanilla extract

8 ounces (225 g) cream cheese 1 cup (11O g) chopped pecans

Mix together all dry ingredients in a large bowl. Blend eggs with a fork, addoil, and blend again. Add the dry ingredients and mix with whisk till smooth. Add and blend in buttermilk, food coloring, and vanilla. Pour into 3 greased and floured 8-inch (20 cm) cake pans. Bake at 350°F (180°C, gas mark 4) for 30 minutes. Cool for 10 minutes and gently remove from pan. To make icing, mix ingredients until light and fluffy. Frost cake when cool.

Yield: 16 servings

Each with: 23 g water; 457 calories (39% from fat, 6% from protein, 55% from carb); 7 g protein; 20 g total fat; 6 g saturated fat; 9 g monounsaturated fat; 4 g polyunsaturated fat; 65 g carb; 3 g fiber; 49 g sugar; 137 mg phosphorus; 40 mg calcium; 1 mg iron; 63 mg sodium; 184 mg potassium; 317IU vitamin A; 85 mg vitamin E; 0 mg vitamin C; 53 mg cholesterol

47 Brown Rice Pudding

This quick rice pudding recipe uses leftover rice. (I tend to make a lot ofrice when I cook it so I can use it in all these recipes calling for leftovers.)

2 cups (44O g) cooked brown rice1½ cups (C55 ml) skim milk

½ cup (17O g) honey

1 cup (145 g) golden raisins 1 tablespoon unsalted butter1 teaspoon cinnamon

In medium saucepan, combine rice, milk, honey, and raisins and bring to boil. Reduce heat and simmer 20 minutes, stirring frequently. Remove from heat and stir in butter and cinnamon.

Yield: 4 servings

Each with: 168 g water; 426 calories (8% from fat, 7% from protein, 85% from carb); 8 g protein; 4 g total fat; 2 g saturated fat; 1 g monounsaturated fat; 0 g polyunsaturated fat; 96 g carb; 4 g fiber; 60g sugar; 235 mg phosphorus; 174 mg calcium; 2 mg iron; 66 mg sodium; 543 mg potassium; 277 IU vitamin A; 80 mg vitamin E; 3 mg vitamin C; 9 mg cholesterol

48 Cool Rice

This is a kind of instant rice pudding and similar to the dish served at many family get-togethers during my childhood.

½ pound (225 g) brown rice

6 ounces (17O g) nondairy whipped topping, such as Cool Whip

¼ cup (5O g) sugar

1 teaspoon vanilla extract

1O ounces (284 g) crushed pineapple 5 maraschino cherries, halved

Cook rice according to package directions and cool.

Yield: 5 servings

Each with: 106 g water; 217 calories (33% from fat, 4% from protein, 63% from carb); 2 g protein; 8 g total fat; 5 g saturated fat; 2 g monounsaturated fat; 0 g polyunsaturated fat; 35 g carb; 1 g fiber; 22 g sugar; 72 mg phosphorus; 50 mg calcium; 0 mg iron; 47 mg sodium; 132 mg potassium; 257 IU vitamin A; 63 mg vitamin E; 4 mg vitamin C; 26 mg cholesterol

49 Whole Wheat Piecrust

I find this oil-based piecrust easier to work with than with solid shortening. And it seems to stay flaky through more handling.

cu⅓ (8O ml) canola oil

1 cups (16O g) whole wheat pastry flour 2 tablespoons (28 ml) water, cold

Add oil to flour and mix well with fork. Sprinkle water over and mix well. With hands press into ball and flatten. Roll between 2 pieces of waxed paper. Remove top waxed paper, invert over pan, and remove other paper. Press into place. For pies that do not require a baked filling, bake at 400°F (200°C, gas mark 6) until lighted browned, about 12 to 15 minutes.

Yield: 8 servings

Each with: 6 g water; 150 calories (56% from fat, 7% from protein, 37% from carb); 3 g protein; 10 g total fat; 1 g saturated fat; 6 g monounsaturated fat; 3 g polyunsaturated fat; 15 g carb; 2 g fiber; 0 g sugar; 69 mg phosphorus; 7 mg calcium; 1 mg iron; 1 mg sodium; 81 mg potassium; 2 IU vitamin A; 0 mg vitamin E; 0 mg vitamin C; 0 mg cholesterol

50 High-Fiber Piecrust

This is a really simple piecrust with 4 grams of fiber. You can add sugar or other sweeteners or spices like cinnamon depending on the final flavor you want.

1 cup (60 g) lightly sweetetened bran cereal, such as Fiber One

½ cup (120 ml) water, approximately

Crush cereal to a powder in a resealable plastic bag. Add any sweetener or spice desired to taste here and shake together. Pour evenly into a 9-inch (23 cm) springform or pie plate. Drizzle a little water at a time just to moisten the crumbs. Spread and press crust evenly. Use as stated in recipe, either baking before or simply pouring filling in and then baking or refrigerating.

Yield: 8 servings

Each with: 15 g water; 15 calories (8% from fat, 7% from protein, 85% from carb); 1 g protein; 0 g total fat; 0 g saturated fat; 0 g monounsaturated fat; 0 g polyunsaturated fat; 6 g carb; 4 g fiber; 0 g sugar; 38 mg phosphorus; 25 mg calcium; 1 mg iron; 27 mg sodium; 45 mg potassium; 3 IU vitamin A; 0 mg vitamin E; 2 mg vitamin C; 0 mg cholesterol

CPSIA information can be obtained
at www.ICGtesting.com
Printed in the USA
BVHW070044270621
610451BV00003B/629

9 781802 895643